COVID Set My Soul On Fire

Danielle Red Owl

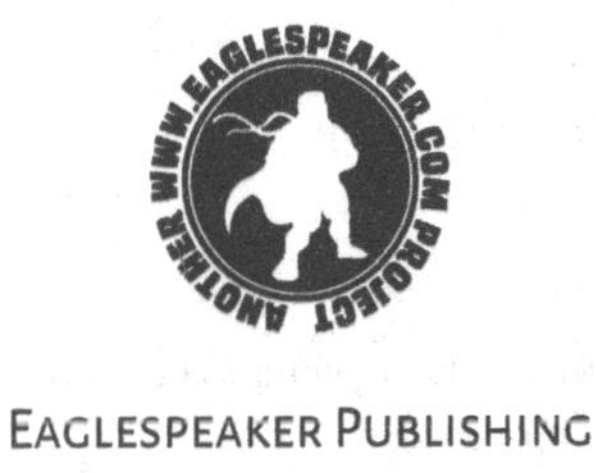

Eaglespeaker Publishing

CONTENTS

In memory of the victims and survivors of COVID-19.

Thank you to all healthcare workers and frontline workers.

To my friends and family, thank you for your encouragement and support.

Acknowledgements

Thanks to the hospital staff at Bryan Health. Thank you to Azria Healthcare for helping me get home. Special Thanks to Michelle Foster and Janet Alesna for helping me reach my goal and being my biggest cheerleaders. Thank you to Angels Healthcare, Bryan LifePointe, CHI Health, UNMC, Psychotherapy and Associates, Morningside Counseling and Madonna Rehabilitation for the therapy services.

Thank you to my dad, Danny Red Owl, for being by my side and making difficult decisions on my behalf. Thank you to my little brother, Devin Henry, for the work on my house to make it handicap accessible. Thank you, Christine Bickerstaff, for raising funds and taking care of my house and puppies. Thank you to my nephew, Beau Red Owl Jr., for taking care of Wrigley and Fenway and all you do for our family.

Thank you to Mark Holbrook for being the best employee advocate. Thank you, PayPal, for supporting me through my COVID-19 ordeal and giving me the opportunity to be a member of the PayPal family.

Thank you, St. David's Episcopal Church and members, for your prayers of encouragement, flowers, gifts and well wishes.

Thank you to Roberta Engstedt and Shelly Avery for being my biggest supporters. Thank you to Paula Johnson and Don Whipple for everything.

Thank you to the Santee Sioux Nation and Ponca Tribe of Nebraska.

Thank you to my Jack's Bar family for your generosity and thoughtfulness.

Thank you to Joan Casey, Stephanie Fitzler and all the generous donors for the GoFundMe account.

Thank you to Becky Busboom for all you do.

Thank you to Jessica Simons for your generous donation.

Thank you to Tommy Arsiaga and Southside Boxing Gym.

Thank you to my medical team: Dr. Kevin Reichmuth, Dr. Carlos Calisto-Perez, Dr. Gerard Haffner, Dr. Amy Garwood, and Dr. Lisa Peterson

Thank you to Erin Marra for book review and recommendations.

Thank you to Jason Eaglespeaker and Eaglespeaker Publishing.

PREFACE

Since my early twenties, I have always wanted to write an autobiography or novel. I would often write short stories for English classes, and I even dabbled in poetry here and there. I found my writing to be honest, real, and authentic in storytelling. At the time, I thought my circumstances were extraordinary, unique, special and a once-in-a-lifetime story of survival and growth, with wisdom beyond my years. However, my childhood experiences were far from spectacular or unique; in retrospect, it is how you endure and forge forward that is truly amazing.

I realized, over time and experience, there are two types of people in the world: the "doers" and the "talkers." The talkers in my definition do just that: they talk. No action is ever taken and can often be identified with statements such as "I need to," "I should," "I could have," "I should have," or "One day..." The talkers "talk the talk" and never "walk the walk." Their statements are often followed up with a long line of excuses on why they could not or did not walk the walk. I would talk a big game about writing an autobiography, often saying "I am going to write a book." Some of my favorite excuses back then were "I'm too busy," "I had to focus on school," "I don't have time." Honestly, I was too caught up partying and never took one single step of action or penned one line toward my book. I learned that if I did not make time, I would never have time.

Today, I pride myself on being a doer. It has taken twenty years and counting to mold myself into a prideful doer. A doer "walks the walk." They can tell you what they are doing and never have to tell you their intentions again; you can follow their actions towards achieving their goal. They aren't afraid of failure and they certainly don't conjure up excuses or use vocabulary such as "I can't" or "I couldn't." They also take full accountability and ownership and simply "just do the damn thing."

I will take you through a rough and tumble battle of survival from beginning to current day and how I overcame the odds to live long enough to tell you about it, laced with authenticity, wit and humor. I'm not a saint, expert, nor a great novelist but I can share with you how my experience spent in an alcoholic home forced me to adapt and survive. My journey to this point in my life has been epic and the lessons learned are incomparable. This is a true story of survival and having the determination and resilience to change my circumstances and how battling COVID-19 set my soul on fire.

CHAPTER ONE

OLD FASHIONED

The life and upbringing I were given is far from ordinary or conventional. I'm not sure that I'm made for the world we live in today. I am a bit of an old soul - I have always emulated the characteristics of my grandparents who grew up during the Great Depression and the Dust Bowl era where harsh circumstances formed people with a greater sense of responsibility. Their work ethic, loyalty, honesty, respect, frugality, integrity and humility are unmatched by any generation since or yet to come.

My grandparents were steadfast in their Christian faith, patriotism, and family traditions. My grandfather fought in World War II, and he was a strong, silent, and humble man. His eyes told a story that he had seen war and more of the world than he would ever be willing to tell me. He believed that my ears were not meant to hear war stories. He had a strong stature; his hands were large, wrinkled, strong, and no stranger to dirt or hard work. He was a man of sturdy character and, although a man of few words, his deadpan humor was epic: he was always telling a joke or saying the funniest thing at the perfect moment. In retrospect, he also had what we now call great "dad-humor." *Such as "what did the dad tomato say the baby tomato? Ketchup."* My grandpa was my guardian angel, my rock, my protector, my father figure who took me into his home every time I needed one.

My grandmother was a bit feisty, and you could tell that she had lived a full life and experienced a lot. Her hands were aged but soft and beautiful and not afraid of work. It was a thing of grace and art to watch this woman cook and her smile was infectious. She also had a mean streak, and I could tell when she was unhappy, whether it was crumpling up her newspaper, or a look, or a sigh of disdain. We had a good relationship, but we did not become close until I moved home to be with her after my grandpa passed away.

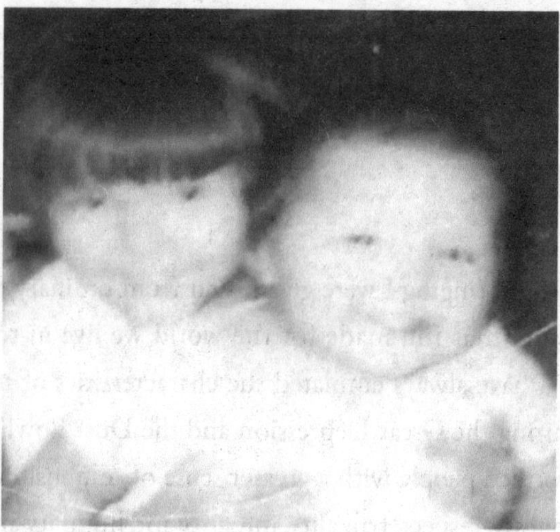

Figure 1: My brother and me

I used to carry a heavy heart, not understanding how my parents could walk the earth and not have our (my brother and I) interests first and foremost. Naïvely, I thought that was what a parent was supposed to do: put their kids first and protect them. But my parents were young and broken with trauma, life, experience, marriage, divorce, heartbreak, and grief, and they did not know how to be the parents we needed.

Eventually, my brother and I both went to live with Grandma and Grandpa, but they continually sent me back to live with my mom. I never understood why until later in life. If anything, I learned how I didn't want to be, and I did not want to put my children through what I went through as a child from a broken, alcoholic, and abusive home. I don't blame my parents; they were married and divorced before I could even remember. I got to know them better in my adult years and learned that they had to grow and find their own path and heal on their own over time. In the end, I came out to be one of the most adaptable, resilient people on the planet, and I love that about me.

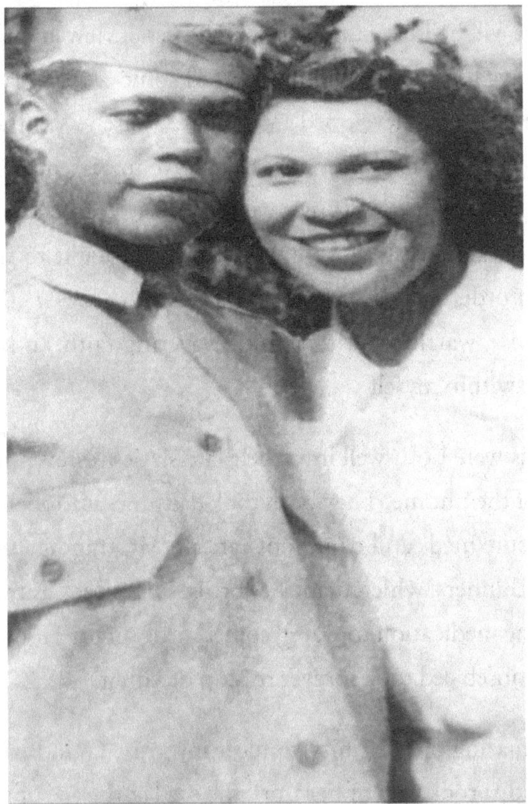

Figure 2: My grandparents in the 1940s

I credit my upbringing to my grandparents because they taught me my greatest life lessons: love, kindness, respect, generosity, humility, faith, and most important of all, forgiveness. I lived with my grandparents off and on throughout my childhood until seventh or eighth grade, when I went to live with them for good. I sometimes wondered if my time with them was but a dream. Then I reminded myself that a bond as strong as we shared with love and laughter cannot be broken and it was not a dream, but a life that was lived and loved. I think that I received the best parts of them-they showed me who I wanted to be in life. Even if they did not birth me, we had that special parent-child bond, and I would be loved and protected by them for eternity.

I could go into the oppression of my Native American people and how genocide and reservation life has adversely impacted me, my parents, and grandparents, but I won't, because that would be a different, longer book. However, there are some things that will help you understand my overall view and thought-process, and how my views formed over the years; and some were already a part of my fundamental being. I have developed a very acute awareness of the type of person I am and the underlying characteristics that drive my essence. I was born with a protective spirit and I protect my loved ones with ferocity and fearlessness. My Native American ancestors were warriors who fought to survive genocide and atrocities in order to keep our relatives on *kuns'i maka*[1]. I find that same resilient, relentless, warrior spirit, with unwavering faith, to keep living for a greater purpose, within myself.

My grandparents were both well into their late sixties to seventies by the time I was in and out of their home. They both took daily medication; my grandpa took high blood pressure meds and could not eat salt. My grandma had diabetes and also took blood thinners, which made her bruise and bleed easily. Blood thinners were a frightening medication to watch someone be on for a long period of time. A simple cut or nosebleed took forever to stop bleeding.

I also had the amazing opportunity to meet my great-Grandma, my Grandpa's mom. My Grandpa took care of her until she died at the age of ninety-eight. All of my grandparents were scared to be taken away from their families and put in a nursing home or hospital. They were adamant that they would never want to be put in a home. I never really understood it until now. Nursing homes never existed in our culture; we were used to taking care of our own people in our community and tribe. My grandparents and other elders in the community were afraid of being mistreated or going there to die, because that is what usually happened in those places. My grandparents never said it out loud, but we were a minority race, and the nearest nursing home was in a white community a town or two over.

My grandparents were of the era of children who were taken away from their families and homes and sent to Indian boarding schools, beaten if they spoke in their native language, and forced to assimilate to white culture. A lot of children never came home, and horrible atrocities happened to many of them, including rape, physical abuse, and even death. All of my grandparents were fluent in the Dakota language, but we no longer spoke it in our house-only in church, where it was permitted to sing Dakota hymns. We were members of the Episcopal Church brought to our reservation by missionaries who translated English hymns, which were played to piano music, and sung in the Dakota language, such as "Amazing Grace," "Sweet By and By," "Rock of Ages," etc. My favorite hymn to sing in the Dakota language is "Sweet By and By"-- I'm not fluent in *Dakodiapi*[2], but I can sing and understand a lot of it.

I believe personalities form at a young age because I have always been an optimist and had a fearless, adventurous way about me. I have never felt satisfied or complete, like I was destined for more. I have been searching and trying to change my circumstances by overcoming overwhelming odds since birth, knocking down barrier after barrier, even the barriers I put in my own way.

I am of the #MeToo population. I was molested when I was five or six while staying at a relative's house when my parents were out partying. I was almost abducted in the fifth grade on my way home from school in the city. I was almost raped in the sixth grade by a relative's boyfriend. I watched a friend of mine die in front of me after being beaten by her boyfriend.

I can attribute almost every traumatic event in my life due to alcohol in some way or another. Most of my childhood was spent in an alcoholic home that was emotionally abusive. A lot of my adolescence was spent moving around to different towns or staying with different relatives. As a result, I gained courage, learned survival traits and developed adaptability at a young age. I kept track of where I lived and who I lived with by what school grade I was in at the time.

My first glimpse of my resilient, unbound determination showed up when I was in the sixth grade. The year prior, when I was in the fifth grade, my mother and I moved off the Santee Sioux Indian reservation and into the city. My mom was drinking heavily by this time, and we moved across town and to a new school. This was our third move within the city in our short time there. Middle school in the city started in the sixth grade, whereas back home it started in the seventh grade. I was bullied at the new middle school and found it hard to make friends there.

I didn't like going to that school, so I rarely attended, and my mom never made me go. I had grown accustomed to doing what I wanted by that time. I missed so much school that I was declared truant, and they sent a case worker to my house to knock on the door about once a week or so. We never answered the door, and my mom helped me move the TV upstairs so the case worker wouldn't hear me watching it during the day. I was extremely smart, and I actually liked school, but I didn't know how to deal with being bullied and the extreme culture shock of being in the city. I attended school sometimes just to learn because I loved to learn, or for a hot meal because we often did not have a lot of food at home. On one rare occasion when I went to school in the sixth grade, I saw a flier for a Math Bee. It blew my mind, and inside I was excited thinking, *"I LIKE MATH! What is a Math Bee?"*

When I saw the Math Bee flier, my mind was set. I wanted to compete in that Math Bee. I went up to my teacher after class was over to inquire about the details and how to get signed up. What is the phrase... "Curiosity killed the cat?" Well, curiosity didn't kill the cat, but it deflated the cat, and told her she couldn't participate in the Math Bee because she was never in school. That is what the teacher said when I asked to be entered in the Math Bee. Even at that young age, I was the one that you couldn't say "no" to when I had my mind made up. I negotiated. I agreed to go to school every day leading up to the Math Bee if the teacher would let me participate. She agreed. I held up my part of the deal and I went to school every day (it was only two or three weeks) and got myself a spot in the Math Bee. I was excited, even if I didn't quite know what a Math Bee was, but it sounded like fun. Even when I went to school every day during that time, I never made any friends and kept to myself to hold up my part of the bargain.

My mom invited my grandparents to the city so they could watch me perform in the big Math Bee event. It was somewhat similar to a Spelling Bee where an audience was present, but instead of announcing the word, they put the math problems up on the projector to display for everyone to see what math questions we worked on. I ended up tying for second place and defaulted to third place in that Math Bee; due to the difference in difficulty of the problems missed. The first and second place competitors were from the gifted classes. I didn't even know that they had gifted classes because I hardly went to school. It wasn't a win, but for a girl off the reservation and not in school regularly, I think I did ok. I was proud of my third-place win-I still am, but I no longer have my ribbon, only the memory.

Looking back, I'm not even sure why that Math Bee was so important, or why I wanted to do it so badly; I just really loved math, I guess. A week or two after the Math Bee, I didn't see my mother for a few days, and I was left at home with no food, no money, and no parent, which became a regular occurrence. I had had enough--I called my grandpa to come get me and he was there the next day to rescue me. I went back to the reservation to live with my grandparents and finished sixth grade there.

My mom eventually followed me to my grandparents' house and, once she got her own house again, I was forced to go live with her; by this time, I was in Jr. high school. I started to drink and smoke; I thought I was the cool kid. I had house parties with my friends, and my mom didn't care and even bought me alcohol and cigarettes. Then one day, in my eighth-grade year, my mom broke into the gas station and stole beer, cigarettes, food, pop, and candy. I didn't want anything to do with it because I knew that theft and burglary was morally wrong and told her so. I went to school the next morning and, sure enough, they knew it was someone in my household. The cops brought my mother to the school to question me because they couldn't question me without a parent present. She put all the blame on me and told the cops that I broke into the gas station. When the cops left the room, she panicked and told me that I had to take the blame for her because she would go to prison, and I would only get probation or go to juvenile detention. When I refused, she started going on about how I would be in a group home, and no one wanted me, and I would be an orphan. The barrage of threats and abuse went on and on. I kept a stoic face and played along, not letting her or anyone know the profound impact that her words had on me and my ability to trust people. I didn't admit to anything; I didn't answer questions with a straight answer. My mom would not leave me alone or allow me to go to court alone. She sat in the courtroom every day while I was on trial for her crime. I thought that surely no one would allow their kid to take the fall for them-the parent is supposed to protect their children. The county attorney even mentioned multiple times that he had thought I was covering up for my mother. Well, that whole "without a doubt" theory of mine went right out the window. I was convicted of felony burglary in the juvenile court system. My Grandpa arranged for my teachers to be character witnesses for me at the sentencing hearing so the judge would not send me to juvenile detention. I was sentenced to probation and was released to my grandpa. I walked right past my mom, looked at my grandpa and said, "I'm coming to live with you from now on," and he agreed. I never went back to live with my mom again. I had probation for a year with a strict curfew where I had to be in my yard by 8 PM every night. It was a good thing we had a big yard and a basketball hoop to keep me busy.

Eventually, my mom followed me to my grandparents' home again but by that time she was vengeful, and even more verbally and emotionally abusive, so much that I just stopped going home. I stayed mostly with friends and relatives, not knowing where I was going to sleep or eat. Thankfully, I had some really great friends and relatives who never made me go home and let me stay with them. My Grandma was not happy that I was hardly home, and I think she might have believed my mom and thought I had done the crime. My Grandpa and I just kind of knew that it was best for me to have space, so he didn't make me go home or come looking for me or mind if I kept his pickup truck for days at a time. He trusted me and could sense I needed to be away from my mom. We only talked about it one time: I wanted to go back to court and have my mom sent to prison-they couldn't do anything worse to me, I already did my time-but he talked me out of it. My Grandpa knew without me telling him that I didn't do the burglary and he would defend me, always, no matter what, before and after that ordeal.

I did everything in my power to get out of the house early and head to college. I took double the math and science, which put me with the upperclassmen. I thought I was one of the coolest nerds you would ever meet, super smart and very laid back. I would help the upperclassmen with homework in math or science and became great friends with most, if not all, of them; I still talk to them today. When eleventh grade rolled around, I was on track to graduate early-I just needed to commit to one summer class for the 2.5 credit hours that I was short. I was onboard but there was one major problem that backfired on me: I never ran my plan by my grandpa, and he was set in his traditional ways. Grandpa said "no" because he thought I was too young. I would have only been sixteen years old if I graduated early, and seventeen later in the fall.

I came up with a backup plan that was not very well-thought-out. I moved with my aunt to Lincoln, Nebraska, hoping to graduate there. I was young and naïve and did not foresee the major flaw in my backup plan that would have saved us all a lot of time: Grandpa had said no, and she was not going to defy her father.

I attended Lincoln High School in 1995, the same year that Teen Magazine visited the high school and the Nebraska Husker football team went to the Orange Bowl. I learned a lot in my short time in Lincoln, mostly how to better cope with culture shock. I went from a class size of six to a class size of about four-hundred to five-hundred students. It wasn't hard to make friends because I had a cousin that lived there who was in the same grade, and she helped me transition in school by introducing me to people. Plus, I had friends that used to live in Santee and had been in Lincoln for some time.

I literally couldn't comprehend why no one would let me graduate. I was so ambitious and ready to be out of my house and on to college. Besides, it wasn't like I was learning much in school by that time because I had already taken everything. My class schedule looked like: homeroom, career survival, study hall, band, the first half of advanced literature, lunch break, the second half of advanced literature, study hall, study hall and some science class. I didn't know what I was supposed to be studying during study hall, so I stopped going to those. I had older friends who would come pick me up from school, so I would run errands or hang out with them for most of the day and be back to the school in time for my aunt to pick me up at the end of the day. My friend had something to do one day and couldn't come get me, so I told my aunt that I didn't want to go to school because they didn't have anything for me to study. Maybe they should have had part-time school back then, for people like me. My aunt made me go to school, so I went. I attended all of the classes on my schedule but when I arrived at my first of three study hall classes, I checked in at the desk and when they found my name, they said I could no longer attend study hall. It caught me by surprise and I had to ask for clarification,

"So, you are kicking me out of study hall?"

After I got an affirmative answer, I asked if she could check her list again because I had two more study halls that day. Yep, I was kicked out of all three study halls due to lack of attendance. I got a hold of my friend and they came to pick me up.

That was the beginning of the end of my stay in Lincoln. I didn't mind the other classes-I enjoyed band class. I used to play the trumpet and it was a big year for band because our marching band was going to the Orange Bowl to cheer on the Huskers. Now, I was young and didn't recall our marching band having uniforms back home in Santee; at least, I had never seen one. One day, I went to band class and they laid out red, white and black polyester uniforms with weird hats and instructed us to pick out our uniform size. I told the band teacher that there was no way I was wearing that. The teacher responded that if I didn't wear the uniform, I could no longer be in the band. I still refused and was kicked out of band as a result. In retrospect, not only did I think I was too cool for the uniform but I was also body-conscious and didn't want to have to pick out my size in front of the entire band. I got into more trouble and moved home to Santee with my grandparents.

I graduated from Santee High School in 1996 with my original class at the age of seventeen, with five other classmates. My mom had me kicked out the week after graduation-I stopped going home and she lied to my grandparents telling them I had been partying. I was just trying to avoid her abuse, not wanting to let it escalate or worsen since my grandpa had talked me out of sending her to prison.

After I was kicked out, I moved in with friends and partied for three months straight. Then, one day my grandpa showed up out of nowhere and rescued me again, this time without me calling him. I don't know how he found me-we didn't have cell phones then-but he was sitting in his car smoking his cigarettes, patiently waiting for me. Once I went outside of the apartment to greet him, he simply said, "It's time to come home now; you have school starting." I rarely defied my grandpa, if at all, so I gathered up what little belongings that I had and went back home with him to start college at the Nebraska Indian Community College in Santee.

It wasn't all bad times with my parents: we had lots of great memories and good times as well. My mom would hold me until I fell asleep when I was sick or stroke my temple to relax me so I would go to sleep on sleepless nights. In the beginning, she was very smart and loving and had a good sense of humor, and she always wanted to be a friend to people. Somewhere along the way, she got lost in alcohol and turned into someone I didn't recognize or care to know. She went through treatment a few times and we eventually had a good relationship. She would call me on my birthday every year, no matter what and I got accustomed to those conversations-I miss them the most. My mom died in 2017 from long-term illness due to a hemorrhagic stroke in 2012.

My brother and I lived with my dad and his mom when we were really little; I may have been between two and four years old. My dad would lie awake sometimes with my brother on one arm and me on the other and listen to the radio to fall asleep. To this day, I still listen to the radio when I sleep. In our small village, my mom's parents were our neighbors. My dad bundled us up and took us next door before his shift at the factory located nine miles outside of the village. It was so early in the morning that it was still dark outside and the stars were bright. The factory closed down and they gave the workers the option to work at another location 120 miles south, in Columbus, Nebraska. My dad remarried and moved away to keep his job, and my brother and I went to live with our mom or other relatives. He would take the two of us for a few weeks in the summer sometimes and to the movies on some holidays: we would see him every Christmas. My dad has been to every one of my graduations. We have gotten to know each other more since I became an adult, and we have grown together to form a close relationship. I can talk to him about anything and I feel at home when I am with him.

I believe that we are connected deeply to our parents, siblings and grandparents, with or without knowing it. I see my grandparents in my aunts, uncle, my brother, and myself. I have my mom's beautiful smile, and my grandparents' values and mannerisms. I have my dad's sense of style with hats and shoes-our fitted hat size is the same. I have seen kids in movies practice forging their parents' names, but I never did that and never knew what my dad's signature looked like. In 2017, I was astonished when I found out that we have almost identical signatures. We submitted land lease transfer paperwork and he thought he had signed the wrong paper and then realized it was my signature and not his. We also have the same sense of humor, and are both very prideful people who would rather go without than ask for help.

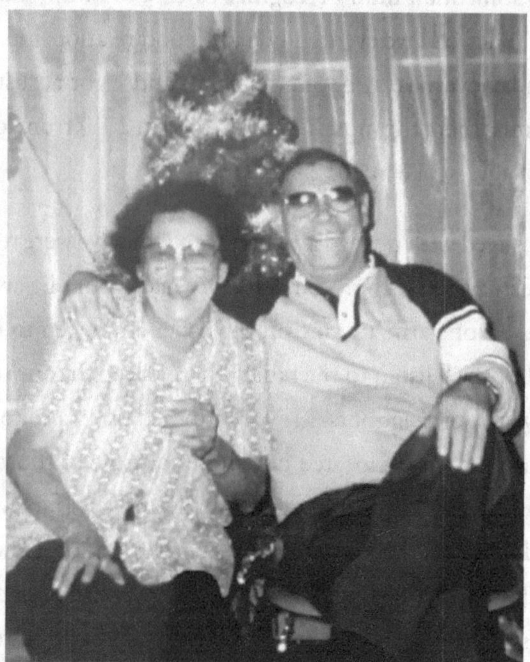

Figure 3: My grandparents in the 1990s

My Grandpa passed away in his sleep from a massive heart attack seventeen months after he brought me home for college. I was clueless about age, time and death. I thought my grandpa and grandma would be in my life forever. When my grandpa died, my foundation crumbled. I lost my faith. I went through a very dark time in my life for two and a half years and lived recklessly, like I had a death wish. I never thought I would live to see thirty. It was during those two and a half years that I helped take care of my grandma. She pulled me out of that dark time. She was the one who slowly restored my faith by showing me her strength, courage, love and unwavering faith. If I thought my grief was extreme, I couldn't imagine what she was going through. I tried my best to be strong for her. I moved away in 2000 and there was not a single day that went by where I didn't call and talk to my grandma. She passed away in 2002. I miss her warmth, love, and our daily conversations the most.

My grandparents both still come to visit and check in on me in my dreams from time to time, and it's as if no time had passed, like it was yesterday. I also see them almost every day in my own mannerisms or within my aunts' and uncle's features, laughter or gestures. My grandparents were such good people. I'm "old school" like Grandma and Grandpa and I love that about me.

CHAPTER TWO

THE CHRONIC

Living with my grandparents was an adventure in itself, and I often got to travel with them. On one road trip from Nebraska to Wisconsin, I remember riding in the backseat with my older brother and playing car games like "ABCs," or "I-spy." We must have been ten or twelve years old, and we knew how to entertain ourselves by using our environment to locate items or count animals that we passed by, when that failed, we would fight. On this particular trip, I had the most excruciating pain in my knees that hurt so much that I began to cry. My tough-love grandparents, who lived and fought through war, diagnosed me with "growing pains." It was my understanding that growing pains occur when the body outgrows the bones, creating a growth spurt in the bones or joints that cause pain. Their diagnosis meant that I was to suffer in silence because it was just a part of life. I sat through that car ride in immense pain and only received relief when we stopped to stretch, get gas, or finally arrived after our ten-to-twelve-hour car ride. That same pain became familiar and haunted me later in life.

I was always active and played sports most of my life; I was the catcher in little league. I don't ever remember being thin, and I was a little heavier than most kids my age, but nothing extreme. I was stocky and strong. I had to be because I had to fend for myself at a young age and had an older brother who would use me as a punching bag to practice his new taekwondo moves on. I have always been scrappy, so I listened and learned; I got my taekwondo lessons for free, and it fed that fearlessness that already lived within my being.

When I was fifteen, I played fastpitch women's softball for the neighboring town team since our village was too small to have its own. My classmate's mom would pick me and my cousin up and take us with her to practice and games in towns within Knox County, Nebraska. It was a fun and happy time to get out of the house to be a part of a team and have something to do in the hot days of Nebraska summer. The age limit to play town sports league was sixteen, but the teammate who picked me and my cousin up for league that summer didn't mind bending the rules-I was only fifteen but all the other kids in my class were already sixteen and besides, I would turn 16 in October. Most people assumed that I was older than my age throughout my entire adolescence and into my early twenties-likely because I hung out with a crowd three to four years older than me.

At my grandparents' house, there was a basketball hoop on a sparse, grassy area in the corner of our large backyard that butted up against the cornfield. Basketball became my brother's primary sport and mine. We would draw a free throw line in the dirt and play "HORSE," "Around the World," or "21." We would play until the sun went down and we could no longer see the hoop, or until we would get into a fight and wrestle each other to the ground.

We were fairly isolated on our side of town because there was a cornfield between us and the main community to the west; and to the north was the main road that went by our house, and beyond that road was the Missouri River that bordered the riverbanks of South Dakota. To the east were a few neighbors, and about four houses down was the local bar. To the south was more of the same cornfield that bordered us to the west. As small as our village was, we had an East and West side of town. We lived a city block or two down from the main East side of town and had to be home before dark. One of our main sources of entertainment in the early '90s (pre-cell phone days) was to walk around town, to and from the West and East sides of town with friends, and still be home by the time the streetlights came on.

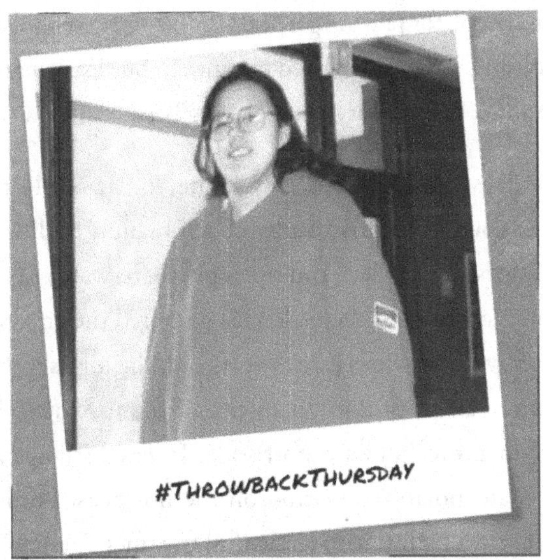

Figure 4: Throwback to Senior Year (1996)

I excelled in basketball in Jr and Sr high school until my senior year when we didn't have enough players to have a girls' basketball team. I took my frustrations out on the court during lunchtime or after school by playing "21" with the boys. I also participated in track and field; I was more of a thrower than a runner by then because my "cool" factor had entered my ego and I thought it was cool to smoke cigarettes.

My stature and grit must have impressed the elderly boxing coach from a couple of towns over. He knew my grandpa and tried to recruit me to join his boxing club. It wasn't popular then for girls to box, so I declined at the time-I had entered the party scene and needed to feed my "coolness" ego. I don't have many regrets in my life, but I do have a few, and that is one of the crossroads that I regret not taking.

After high school, I partied all summer long until the fall when my grandfather came to bring me home so I could start school at the local community college. I had already taken a couple of college classes during the twelfth grade since the high school had run out of subjects for me to take. I hung out with all the college kids and hit the party scene hard. I still managed to get passing grades without much effort. I am sure the professors could tell I wasn't giving my full effort, but my work met the criteria for passing grades. I didn't finish school during that first start at the community college; I partied too much, but I still managed to remain physically active at the community gym, playing basketball and volleyball.

During the holidays, the entire family came to our little three-bedroom doublewide trailer house for Christmas break. Our family tradition was to attend church for Christmas Eve services and open gifts afterward. My grandpa called out the names on each gift and the little kids delivered the gifts to the recipient. On Christmas Eve, when I was eighteen years old, the joints in my hand locked up, and it was extremely painful to do any minimal movement. I couldn't even open or close my hand to hold a can of soda. It was a strange and unfamiliar pain. We lived on an Indian reservation on the northeast border of Nebraska and South Dakota with no immediate medical treatment available, and the local Indian Health Service (IHS) clinic was closed until after the holiday. The nearest hospital was a fifty-five-minute drive. I didn't have a vehicle, and the pain and joint stiffness didn't seem urgent enough to call the IHS ambulance. We also didn't have health insurance and urgent care clinics did not exist then, or, at least, not in our rural area. Similar to the growing pains, I just had to suffer through it. I took some Tylenol and blew it off as we opened our Christmas gifts.

The unwritten rule among my friends was that we would all get together and party Christmas Eve after family time was done. A friend of mine would usually come pick me up or check to see what time I would be ready and come back to get me. That Christmas, I drank the pain away and the joints in my hand unlocked; the pain didn't return when I woke up the next day.

On Christmas Day, my family met one last time for Christmas dinner before they retreated back to the homes that they traveled from. I got my small corner of my grandparents' house back. The joint pain was such an odd occurrence and surely couldn't have been growing pains. I was 5'9" tall and eighteen years old, so I wrote it off as an anomaly without giving it much more thought.

Another year or two passed, and then Christmas came around again with the same family and friend traditions: family first, and then meeting up with my friends to party. That year, it was not my hand joints that locked-it was both of my knees. I was in so much pain that it was unbearable to bend at the knee to sit or stand. I took a ton of ibuprofen and found myself in the same situation as before-there was no medical treatment available unless I called 911 for an ambulance. I must've been nineteen or twenty by then, because I was able to drink in the neighboring town tavern. The pain was so excruciating that I stood the entire night and drank until I could no longer feel pain. The immense pain frightened me because it immobilized my ability to walk or function normally. I knew that it wasn't healthy to take ibuprofen and consume lots of alcohol, but it was either that or curl up into a ball and cry. I thought, "*What good would that do?*" I had lived through some traumatic events before and chose not to develop a victim mentality, so why would I start now?

The following day, I woke up slightly hungover and relieved that the pain in my knees had gone away. I had to drive my brother back to Lincoln, a three and a half hour drive one-way. I was extremely paranoid that the pain in my knees would return, and I wouldn't be able to drive there and back. I recruited one of my friends to drive with me just to be safe. Thankfully, the pain didn't reappear on our trip, but it stayed in the back of my mind. It was a familiar pain. The pain that I felt in my knees when I was younger in our long car ride to Wisconsin was the same type of pain that I felt over the weekend. Although the pain had dissipated and had not returned, it had such an adverse effect on my ability to walk that I made an appointment to go to the IHS clinic. My level of pain tolerance was skewed because of the alcohol and pain meds.

During my visit with the IHS healthcare provider, I described the pain in the knee joints from the most recent weekend and the pain in the hand from the last incident. As I was explaining my concerns, I thought to myself, "*Do I sound crazy? Listen to me, describing pain that arrives and disappears at random.*" The healthcare worker didn't think I was crazy; instead, he listened, and decided to test me for Rheumatoid Arthritis (RA). He explained that RA was common in the Native American female population, and a simple blood draw to test the RA factor would help identify if that could be the problem. We lived in such a rural area that the lab test took about two weeks to be sent out and returned. I agreed and gave my blood.

Two weeks or so had passed and the clinic finally called to make another appointment to discuss the results. When I arrived at the clinic, the healthcare worker explained that in a normal person without RA, the Rheumatoid factor would be in the double digits, something like seven to twenty. The healthcare worker further explained that they thought my test was contaminated because my first RA factor came back in the low 200s. He recommended another blood test, so I obliged. Another two weeks passed, and this time my RA factor came back in the 410-420 range. The healthcare worker was still in disbelief and was convinced the blood test was tainted or false, so we sent a third blood sample. The results on the third test were in the 700s, and they finally accepted that the tests were accurate and diagnosed me with RA. They also advised me that they had never seen RA factor so high and started me on mild treatments with anti-inflammatory drugs and pain medication.

I was angry about having RA. How could I be sentenced to live in pain for the rest of my life, dealing with a chronic illness? Hadn't I suffered enough in this life already? Worst of all, wasn't I too young to have *arthritis*?

In my twenties, I was in denial and carried anger with me about the diagnosis I received for RA so I didn't take my disease seriously. I continued to drink while on potent medications that would spike my liver enzymes. I kept replaying buzzwords from the educational information provided:

"Chronic illness, no cure."

"Debilitating, permanent damage."

"Immune system attacks the joints and organs."

It's like I have *Fight Club* within my body. My immune system is "Tyler Durden" and my joints and impacted organs are "The Narrator," played by Edward Norton. The first rule of fight club is "We don't talk about fight club!" I'm not ashamed or embarrassed about my chronic illness; I simply don't talk about my internal fight club with Rheumatoid Arthritis because I absolutely refuse to let it define me. In fact, most people don't even know that I live with such a debilitating disease, and I never lead with, "Hi, my name is Danielle, and I live with severe Rheumatoid Arthritis." I had some debilitating events throughout my late-twenties and mid-thirties that left me temporarily immobile and damaged my joints, causing me to lose full functionality of my wrists, hands, and knees. I am fortunate to have learned to advocate for myself over the years and have found a medical team that listens to me and values my instincts and input regarding my healthcare and treatment of RA.

Some people say they can smell when the rain or a storm is coming; my superpower is that I can feel when the weather changes through my joint pain.

MAINSTREAM SOCIETY

The last time my RA factor was tested, the results were in the 2,000s. The RA factor is no longer used to diagnose RA, but I imagine I am on my own chart, since they didn't believe the first few tests in the beginning of my RA journey and the latest results seemed astronomical.

Being diagnosed with RA pissed me off and put me in denial for quite a few years, and I didn't take care of myself or my illness. I partied for days on end, lived recklessly and self-medicated my symptoms with alcohol and drugs. It wasn't until I moved from the reservation into mainstream society that I started to take my health seriously.

I was never given the basic tools or knowledge that were needed to gain independence and be self-sufficient in everyday living. The culture shock was overwhelming because I was extremely unprepared. In fact, the first few attempts that I made to relocate from a small reservation to mainstream society as a young adult ended in failure. I always knew the importance of employment and money but never knew stability at home, financially or otherwise. I worked at numerous temporary employment agencies and held several entry level manufacturing positions including cell phone battery assembly, hydraulic press operator, and catalog inserter. I didn't know how to keep up with bills, budget, pay rent or mortgage, utilities, or obtain medical or dental insurance.

In the year 2000, I graduated from the Nebraska Indian Community College, with two associates in general studies, an Associate of Arts and an Associate of Science. I have two general degrees because I needed an elective to graduate; my brother was in Anatomy which was taught by my favorite Science teacher, so that was my elective and it qualified me for the Science Associate. I used to do random crazy stuff like that that interested me. One time, my brother was in a health class and their class was going to a funeral home. It sounded interesting and I thought we were going to see a cadaver, so I jumped in and went with them. We met at the local bar and carpooled to the funeral home a couple towns over.

The teacher asked, "Are you in my class?"

"I am today," I responded.

We never saw any bodies or spooky stuff, but we had a tour of the facility and watched a video on grief.

After graduation, I decided to move back to the city again and packed my suitcases with my renewed determination, to not fail and move back to the reservation like I had done previously. My "why" was bigger this time. I had the foresight to see that the party scene wasn't to be my fate forever. The need to learn, grow, and use my intellect screamed from within. It was at about that same time that methamphetamine had hit hard in my tiny community, and I observed a dynamic shift: the drugs were becoming a way of life instead of a recreational activity and I needed to remove myself from that precarious scene.

The new venture was lonely. I had to leave my friends and family to start over and create a new life for myself in Lincoln, Nebraska. In the first few months on my journey, I failed at the University and ended up working two jobs to pay for my apartment because I had signed a year lease. I was willing to sacrifice my education to remain in the city that I wanted to call my home. I worked part-time at a retail store and full-time at a gas station. The culture shock I endured during this time in my life was alarming. I was extremely unprepared and not equipped with simple knowledge of business casual attire, vacation, or health insurance, but I knew that I needed a job or two to sustain myself to pay rent and utilities.

The next summer after dropping out of the University, I went home and worked. When I returned to Lincoln in the fall of 2001, I started out with a temporary employment agency that I had used in the past, as I was familiar with their ability to find jobs for people like me. The first assignment was to pass out brochures and show passersby the new Chevrolet Avalanche, a newly designed truck that had access to fold the seats down from the truck bed to the cabin. The assignment lasted about a week at the Nebraska State Fairgrounds in Lincoln. (The Nebraska State Fair has since relocated to Grand Island, Nebraska). A job was a job. The assignment was easy and successful and showed the employment agency that I was reliable. I landed a second assignment for ninety days doing data entry at a large insurance company. It got my foot in the door to corporate America. I had never done data entry before, but I passed a typing test with ease and learned extremely quickly. I often joke that I learn like "Trinity" in the blockbuster movie *The Matrix*. When "Neo" asks if she can fly a helicopter, and the training program is downloaded in her mind in a matter of seconds, and with a few flickers of the eyes, she replies, "I can now," then proceeds to fly the helicopter.

Although the data entry assignment was only for ninety days, it had the opportunity to lead to a full-time position. I wanted to be a full-time, permanent employee, not fully understanding what that involved. It could be my first full-time job in mainstream society, and I was more determined than ever to land it. I treated that ninety-day assignment as though my life depended on it. I wanted the client to feel as though they were losing "an asset" at the end of the ninety-day assignment.

The first few weeks in the office, I was extremely self-conscious and embarrassed because the dress code required business casual attire and I didn't know what that meant. I was too embarrassed to ask someone, and I didn't have money to buy new clothes. I showed up with Nike cargo pants, a white t-shirt with a sweater vest over it and brown Nike shoes. (At least they were not high tops or basketball shoes). I was extremely under-dressed and embarrassed, but held it within. I observed what other people were wearing and mixed some of their styles together to form my own business casual style. It took more than a few weeks to build up a wardrobe because I didn't make much money-I think I made $8.16 per hour. I bought one or two items of clothing every pay period until I had enough for a week's worth of outfits.

My wardrobe crisis and culture shock had no bearing on my work ethic and learning ability. I volunteered for everything: weekends, testing new processes, team outings. I had data entry races with myself to beat my own personal best time, so I could be efficient and accurate and maintain high-quality work. I learned on-the-job-I quickly mastered the keyboard shortcuts and could data enter an application without touching a mouse once. I even taught some of the veteran workers the new shortcuts that I had discovered.

It was September 11th, 2001, and I was getting ready to go to work. I was listening to the radio while I got ready when they announced that a plane had crashed into the World Trade Center Tower. At first, I didn't think it was real, so I went and turned on my TV to the news station and watched the live coverage. I had no idea what to do. I was scared, so I called my grandma and talked to her and asked her what I should do. She told me to go to work and that they would let me know what I should do there.

I went to work and arrived in a somber atmosphere. Everyone was shaken up and uncertain on what we were to do. We tried to work as best we could, but often found ourselves huddled around a computer watching live coverage on the internet, or listening to the radio. I huddled behind a supervisor's computer with a group of coworkers that were my friends and watched the live coverage with them. The supervisor turned and looked at me and told me to get back to my desk and get back to work. I thought about that for a long time, because no one else had to return to their desk but me. I wasn't sure if it was because I was the only minority, the only female or if it was because I was a temporary employee or a combination of all three. It was such a frightening situation that happened that I couldn't just sit there while they all stood and watched. I worked for a bit but I joined the huddle again at the risk of being fired or getting into trouble. The world was stunned, but we slowly got back to work while keeping an eye on the news. I didn't get into trouble for watching the news with my coworkers that I was aware of but found it odd that I was singled out like that. I decided to not give any reason for anyone to fire or reprimand me from that day forward and I continued to excel at my data entry job.

At the end of my ninety-day assignment, I applied for a full-time position and was hired on the spot. I sat through my first new employee orientation in corporate America and had no idea what to do with all the benefits and options they offered, so I signed up for all the insurances and all the benefits that were available. I had health insurance, life insurance, and dental insurance, but I didn't know what to do with any of it. I even had a lump sum of vacation days to use from the first day. I had never had vacation before. I worked nearly three months straight without missing a day before I finally asked my supervisor how to take a vacation day.

I had to figure out how to find a doctor and a dentist. Evidently, you look them up from a directory on the health insurance website. I had never had to find a doctor before, so I went into it with an open mind. I decided that I would make an appointment and go meet the doctor to see if I liked them or not. My first attempt to find a doctor didn't go so well. I showed up for my appointment and they asked for my Medicaid card. I didn't have Medicaid and I thought it was stereotypical, so I left, went on down the list and found a different doctor. I had no ailments other than my RA, but I treated the doctor appointments like interviews: I either liked them or I didn't and moved on to the next one until I felt comfortable enough with a doctor who listened. The doctors were surprised by my tactic to find a new doctor, like I was the only person to ever do this "doctor-interview" method. They expected to see a sick person or someone with a medical need, and I just went to meet-and-greet and quizzed them to see if we had good rapport.

After my selection process, I found a primary care physician (PCP) that fit me and accepted my health insurance. It wasn't until my late twenties that I started to take my RA seriously and found a rheumatologist. I was prescribed a slew of medications, including a chemo-based drug called methotrexate. I took more medication to combat the side effects of the chemo-based drug than the good it did for my RA. Most medications for RA suppressed my immune system so it wouldn't attack my body as quickly.

I was on a trial drug called Simponi when I developed a staph infection in my left hand. I was misdiagnosed by urgent care and the emergency room, where both doctors looked at my medical history and noticed I marked RA down and they attributed the unbearable pain to RA. Every time I went to see a doctor, I was prescribed stronger and stronger pain medication. I took so many pain pills. At first, one pill would make me drowsy and put me to sleep. By the end of that first week, I could take two oxycodone and stay wide awake. I took notice of how fast my tolerance to those narcotics increased, so I no longer took the same drug twice in a row and instead rotated them.

In the end, I had to have surgery on my left hand to remove the infection. The surgeon let me know in the consultation that he may have to cut the muscles and tendons as a worse-case scenario. I asked, "Do those grow back?" He was amused by the question but told me "No." Thankfully, he was able to cut out the infection and save the muscles and tendons. Due to the depth of the wound, I wasn't able to take my arthritis medication because it suppressed my immune system, which created higher risk for additional infection and slowed the healing process. I went without my arthritis medications for approximately eight to twelve weeks. During that time, my immune system ran rampant. It attacked my joints aggressively on a daily basis, which caused such excruciating pain that it was a struggle to simply get out of bed. The pain was so severe that I literally had to convince myself to take my "good" arm with the shoulder joint that could move to pull the other shoulder and leg joints out of their locked state.

The survival mentality and pain that I endured every single day during that time was immense, life-changing and depressing. You don't understand the word pain until you have lived through continuous, debilitating pain for eight to twelve weeks with no relief. Every day was like watching the same bad movie over and over that would never end. The pebble bones in my wrists fused together during that time. I also lost partial functionality of both knees. When I returned to the rheumatologist, to discuss going back on arthritis medication, he advised that I only had one option and that was to go on an infusion medication called Remicade. One of the side effects of that drug was death. I have never liked ultimatums or being backed into the corner. *"Nobody puts Baby in the corner."*

That experience taught me to advocate for myself and for my health, something I had never done before. It also made me reluctant to write my medical history down, so new doctors would assess me and not just attribute any little pain to my RA. I showed him that I did have another option; I decided to get a second opinion. I left that rheumatologist and never looked back. I met my new and current rheumatologist in 2012. My new doctor not only listened but laid out my options for me in a way that I understood them with no bullshit. To this day, she has never backed me into a corner to tell me I have no other options. She tells me that I am at the "top of the drug food chain but there are options-limited options, but options."

I have been through the thick of it with my RA that I dubbed "Baby Arthur" over the years. I am a kid at heart, and love humor so I call my fight with arthritis "The Epic Battle between "Baby D" (my alter ego) versus Baby Arthur." Over time, I learned that the chemo-based drug didn't work for me; it did more damage than good, and I still partied then, which caused my liver enzymes to be elevated. I also discovered that most drugs that I would be on for the rest of my life had the risky side effect of "death." I always joke and say, "I hope I don't get that one (death)!" Some of the medications wiped out my immune system for five years at a time. If I stopped taking my medication today, it would still take my immune system up to five years to fully recover. The true severity of my RA amazes me and scares the crap out of me at the same time. I'm fortunate to still have my own original joints and the ability to walk.

The debilitating hand surgery that I endured motivated me to get involved in the fight with RA. The Arthritis Foundation of Nebraska hosted an annual Walk to Cure Arthritis in May and I created a team named "Baby D's Wolfpack" to raise funds for the cause. It started in 2012 and I sold team t-shirts and hosted an Indian Taco Sale to raise funds and have participated in the walk for several years since.

The fact that the potency of the drugs I am on takes so long for my immune system to recover is indicative of how severe my RA is and how weak my immune system needs to be to maintain a balance between pain, daily living, and independence. Over the years, I have become keenly aware of germs and the impact on my health with my suppressed immune system. I joke a lot about my health and add witty humor to the updates in the "Epic battle between Baby D vs. Baby Arthur." Humor is a healing art, at least in my case.

I used to say that I am a hypochondriac and germaphobe, which has some truth. One time, a lady sneezed on me, and you should have seen the look on my face- I could have killed her with a glance. I likely would have sneezed right back at her if I knew how to sneeze on command. I wonder if it is scientifically possible to sneeze on command. Yes, I did get sick from whatever germs or viruses she shared with me. I developed anxiety about germs and getting sick because I know that a simple cold in me is ten times worse than a normal person with a functioning immune system. Living with RA is extremely hard to describe to someone who doesn't understand that my immune system attacks itself and causes daily, continuous pain. The pain is always there but I am a master of distraction and never focus on it. I manage to live and function daily with managed RA and manageable pain.

Twenty-plus years of living with RA has allowed me to be an astute advocate for my health and well-being. I turned forty on Oct 2, 2018. What a week that was. I ended up getting shingles that week. Happy Fucking Birthday! I advanced to biologic drugs which were infused every six months. I was on Rituxan, which basically wiped out my white blood cells in two-dose infusions, two weeks apart. I was still drinking on the weekend or whenever I had pool or dart leagues, but my partying days had decreased significantly over the years.

On the morning of my fortieth birthday, I received the best birthday gift to date: my nephew messaged me and wanted to come live with me. I had taken him school-shopping earlier that fall and let him know that I would come get him anytime he wanted to come live with me. It was a coincidence that my dad was coming to Lincoln that week for a business meeting and to help celebrate my birthday. I called my dad and arranged for him to pick up my nephew the next morning. I told my nephew that Grandpa would be outside the next morning. My brother also came, and I was happy to see them. He stayed with us for a while and he was my new drinking buddy. We went out mostly on the weekend or sometimes during the week. It was nice to have someone around that could help fix things and help with the handy work.

I tripped and fell after celebrating New Year's in 2019 and broke a rib or two. Around the same time, my immune system stepped up its fight game. I had a small one-year-old puppy named Wrigley who had no idea what broken ribs were-he just wanted to play and frequently pounced on me like "Tigger." I had to walk around with a pillow under my shirt for the first two months of the year because Wrigley was fast. In addition, I had developed red patchy areas of skin on my lower legs which my PCP thought was cellulitis and started me on antibiotics. I ended up being on antibiotics for about a month or three. I sensed that something was wrong, but I couldn't quite figure it out; I concluded that my immune system was running amok. I had developed a goose egg sized knot in the middle of my shin and my rheumatologist sent me to the Infectious Disease Consultants (IDC) to find out what it was. The diagnosis ruled out some fancy doc terminology, but the final diagnosis was Erythema Nodosum (EN). They do not know the cause of EN, but it could be due to antibiotics, which makes sense. It is my understanding that EN can be caused by an overactive immune system, due to antibiotics, or some other unknown cause. Bottom line: my immune system was overactive, and the antibiotics pissed it off. We stopped the antibiotics immediately and the goose egg on my shin went away on its own over time, but my overactive immune system did not. My doctor calmed my immune system down with a shot of steroids to the bum. Even when facing new illnesses due to my overactive immune system, I have never let my RA define who I am.

CHAPTER FOUR

HELLO COVID

F ast forward to the end of 2019, a new "viral pneumonia" originated in Wuhan, China according to the World Health Organization's website. I watched as what would become known worldwide as COVID-19, aka coronavirus or SARS-CoV-2, spread throughout the world in pandemic fashion.

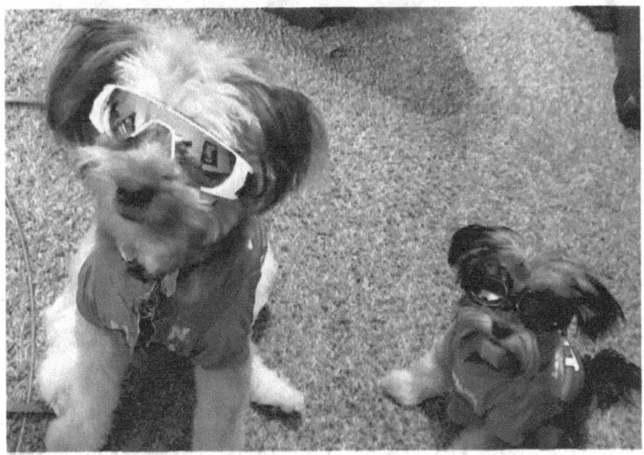

Figure 5: Wrigley and Fenway

Early in 2020, I thought I would be required to return to my office, my nephew would attend school in-person, and our puppy, Wrigley, would be home alone and in need of a playmate. We adopted another puppy on my nephew's eighteenth birthday and named him Fenway. He only knew me and my nephew and hadn't been socialized so he growled and nipped at anyone that came near us because he was overprotective. He also had a hilarious personality, played games, smiled and cuddled, but only for my nephew and me. Fenway was our Sour Patch, COVID baby-both sour and sweet, like the candy commercials.

In late March of 2020, the United States and most of the world went into a pandemic shutdown. It was truly heart-wrenching to watch thousands of people dying at a rate that would require refrigerated trucks to be parked outside the hospitals in metropolis cities to hold all the corpses.

Pre-COVID, I had already evolved into a germaphobe and hypochondriac with an astute sense of personal well-being from living with RA for over twenty years. My compromised immune system, due to the medications that treat RA, caused my anxiety to increase as the pandemic spread.

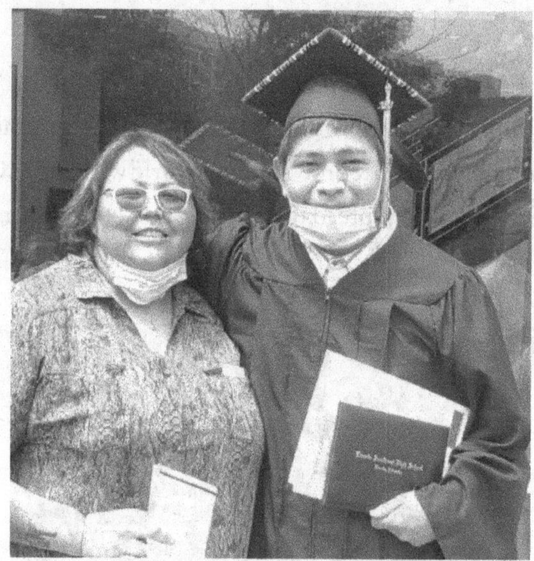

Figure 6: My nephew, class of 2020

Our local community was on lockdown and face masks or coverings were required in public areas. My nephew had to finish his senior year via remote learning. Grades were changed to pass or fail. It was uncertain if Lincoln was going to have graduation ceremonies. However, they were able to organize graduation where six-foot-social distancing was achieved through assigned seating at Pinnacle Bank Arena. We were allotted six tickets per graduate. I was extremely proud of my nephew for successfully transitioning from a rural school of twelve to fifteen students to a class of five hundred or more. He earned his first eagle feather that year, and I taught him how to store it and pray with it. He wore it to graduation on his graduation cap. I was fortunate enough to come up with the funds for his senior pictures and to pay for his graduation reception. I got a crash course in single parenthood and budgeting, but we made it work. He was happy, so I was happy.

I was working as a freelance Senior Business Analyst with contracts for state and federal agencies. I made up to $95k per year, but I paid higher out-of-pocket costs for health insurance, which was quite expensive, and that cut into my net income. Additionally, I did not earn vacation as a contractor, due to the short-term employment agreements. My experience as a freelance business analyst was fun. I met a lot of great people, but I was ready for a change. The pandemic hit hard and most offices were shut down, so we were allowed to work remotely. During that time, I asked myself, *"When was I the most satisfied and successful in my career?"* I determined that I was the most successful and happiest when I worked in large corporations where I felt like I was a part of a family and was making important, progressive changes and contributions to the financial services industry. I loved math and working with numbers. I made innovative and efficient changes to large national financial services institutions and the insurance company that hired me for my first full-time job in corporate America, twenty years ago. I loved having the autonomy to be hands-on and the ability to figure out some of the most complex calculations in the financial industry. I automated or streamlined processes that had provided significant improvement in efficiency for business operations for those companies. I felt needed, accomplished, and well within my element in corporate America. My keen adaptability and survival skills served me well in the business environment. Without rattling off my resume and to shorten up this career ponderance, I decided in early 2020 that it was worth the risk to jump careers and re-enter corporate America where I had previously flourished and made progressive contributions. I wanted to feel like a part of a family with long-term goals and to get away from short-term free-lance contracts.

At the same time, I was still battling an overactive immune system. I had developed red, dry patches areas on my elbows and experienced significant joint pain regardless of the Rituxan infusions. I self-diagnosed myself with Psoriatic

Arthritis (PsA) because of the significant breakthrough joint pain. I went to my PCP and advised that I thought I had PsA. She didn't believe me, but instead thought I had a rash or dry skin. I went to my rheumatologist and told her my suspicions and she sent me to the dermatologist for a biopsy. A few weeks later the biopsy came back and SURPRISE! Psoriasis. I'm not one to say "I told you so," but my instincts are rarely wrong when it comes to self-diagnosing when I am not well. Living with severe RA has taught me to trust my instincts and advocate for my well-being. The biopsy results did not determine if it was regular Psoriasis (PsO) or Psoriatic Arthritis (PsA), but with my joint pain and fatigue, I surmised PsA.

It frightened me to make a career jump during the pandemic because most of the world had shut down and many jobs were lost. I was fortunate to have found a great opportunity with a top-notch organization in the financial services industry whose goals and mission matched mine. I decided to take a job with PayPal, Inc., as a Senior Business Analyst. I took a hit in annual salary by about $17k-$20k but determined it was worth the risk and reduction in gross income for a comparable compensation package and an opportunity to reenter corporate America.

I started my career with PayPal at the end of May 2020. It was a strange experience starting a new job virtually during the pandemic. They shipped me computer, monitors, etc.- everything but the desk and the chair. My main communication with my manager was via text or through Microsoft Teams. I was excited for the new career adventure and enjoyed my team and learning the ins and outs of the job. I was used to working on XML, SQL code and calculations behind the user interface. This job was different. I had to learn to limit my query intel and use limited front-end user interfaces to try to create reports and queries to compute or provide the data I needed to do the job. I was told the learning curve would be about eighteen months; some people may have been intimidated by that time frame but learning is fun for me, especially when it has anything to do with numbers and business analytics.

Honestly, the pay cut was quite an adjustment at first. I was used to having way more expendable cash and had managed to acquire a nice townhome, vehicle and financial stability for myself. Plus, I had my nephew with me now and

I was a parent for the first time in my life. We had no support at all from his parents-financial, emotional, or otherwise. I picked up a second job over the summer writing keno at Cappy's Hot Spot and worked Tuesday through Thursday in the evenings. The pay was less than minimum wage, but the tips made up for it most days. I took the job to replace some of my expendable income that I grew accustomed to when I used to go to the bars regularly. A lot of my friends worked there so it was fun most nights. Plus, it was steady and reliable work, until everything shut down due to the pandemic.

In June 2020, I revisited my Rheumatologist about the biopsy results and we stopped the Rituxan infusions that treated moderate to severe RA. Instead, I started to take Xeljanz which treated both RA and PsA. Rituxan would have long-term lingering effects on my body and immune system for up to five years. Xeljanz was a medication that also suppressed the immune system, like any other RA drug, so my immune system wouldn't attack the joints and body. Xeljanz was one of the first medications in pill form, which was a nice change from the repetitive infusions.

I kept up on the news about the COVID-19 virus, side effects, and its impact on the lungs and risk of going on a ventilator. The risk was fifty-fifty on whether someone would survive being put on the ventilator or if they would succumb to their illness and die. I knew those risk figures were for people with normal immune systems. In my mind, the likelihood for someone like me with little to no immunity surviving intubation was far lower and more like twenty-five percent or less. I was extra cautious and had high anxiety when I was out in public. I carried hand sanitizer with me everywhere I went and wore a mask, as recommended by the experts that were studying this new virus. I started to wear my contact lenses more than my glasses because the mask fogged up my glasses and I was unable to see.

I had a COVID scare in August 2020. I went to my hometown and although everyone around us was not wearing a mask, I made sure to have my mask on at all times. It was after I returned home that I realized people in my small community had tested positive for the new virus. I was in close personal contact with many of them by getting hugs and handshakes, and I was scared that I could have contracted COVID-19. I went to my doctor's office to get tested right away. I got a coworker to cover my shift for my keno-writing job. I also made my nephew attend school virtually just to be safe and waited for the results.

I found it mind-blowing that this little virus traveled all the way from Wuhan, China to find me on an itty-bitty Indian reservation in northeastern Nebraska. Two days after the jab (COVID test) to the brain through my nose with a long Q-tip, the test results were negative. "The masks do work!" I proclaimed to my coworkers and family, and encouraged them to wear a mask and use hand sanitizer at every chance in public. I knew then that catching the virus would mean that I would have a huge fight on my hands because of my compromised immune system. I felt like I had dodged a bullet with the negative COVID test, but I was absolutely convinced that the masks worked.

I worked remotely from home full-time for my day job and there was no risk there. Cappy's placed plexiglass above the keno counter to provide a barrier between us and the customers in order to protect us from the airborne disease. In August, a friend of mine quit drinking and needed sober friends. I decided that, for them, I could be a sober friend. I quit drinking alcohol on August 26th, 2020. I figured, "Why not?" I would save a ton of money and besides, I had started drinking at such a young age-it was time to break the cycle to work on myself and on being a better parent. I was still learning how to be the person for my nephew that I had needed when I was his age.

Little by little, life started to resume. I took my nephew, his friend, and our puppies to Yellowstone National Park over Labor Day weekend. I turned forty-two years old on October 2nd, 2020. I had a small dinner gathering with a couple of friends and my nephew. I attended a fundraiser on October 4th for a friend who had been diagnosed with breast cancer. I played pool league on a Monday night, October 5th, but I had a mild headache. My instincts sensed that I didn't feel quite right, that something was off internally. I stayed away from my pool team and sat at my own table, just to be safe in case I was getting sick.

The very next day, October 6th, I had a prolonged headache; my chest felt heavy; I had a slight cough with an itchy throat, and my muscles cramped. I went to my doctor's office, praying that I had a cold, but my sense of smell was gone too. Deep down, I knew that I had COVID-19. The doctor looked me over, tested me for strep throat, which was negative, and did the COVID test through the nose again. This time he gave me a Z-pack (antibiotics). He told me to quarantine for fourteen days and stop Xeljanz immediately to give my immune system a chance to fight. I went to the pharmacy on my way home and picked up my antibiotics. When I arrived at home, I advised my nephew that I was sure that I had contracted COVID and he should stay home, quarantine, and do remote learning for school and not go to his part-time job. He immediately said, "I think I have COVID also." I sent him to get tested. I then advised my friends and pool team whom I was in close proximity with recently that I thought that I had COVID and that they should be cautious, watch for symptoms, and get tested. Two days had passed, and the results were finally in: **SARS-COV-2 Detected.**

CHAPTER FIVE

FIST FIGHT WITH RONA

My nephew went to the CVS drive-thru to get a COVID-19 test. We assumed that he also had COVID, and we began our quarantine one or two days apart. His test results took a few days and came back positive for COVID-19. I am not sure who gave whom COVID-19, but out of the few people we had encountered during the weekend, we were the only two that ended up with COVID-19. I had only done one thing differently: I walked into a gas station without protective eyewear but wearing a mask. I hypothesized that I had either contracted COVID through the eyes by passing an infected person who had just coughed at the gas station, or I could have forgotten to sanitize my hands before I took my contacts out. There was no way for me to know or track it.

During the first three days of my quarantine, the virus attacked me rapidly, with a massive pressure headache, a heavy chest and severe fatigue. The symptoms were debilitating and prevented me from working and normal daily functions because I could not keep my eyes open. It seemed like I had a cold, but the pressure headaches were extremely intense, blinding and draining. The heaviness in my chest frightened me, as I knew many people who contracted COVID-19 had their oxygen restricted and required supplemental oxygen. Oximeters that measure oxygen level and heart rate were in high demand. I called ahead to the pharmacy to verify that they had some in stock and they confirmed that they had two available.

I advised the pharmacy personnel that I had tested positive for COVID-19 and asked if I had their permission to come through the drive-thru to purchase an oximeter. They told me it was okay and to let them know when I arrived. I was nervous and had anxiety, not because I had COVID-19, but because I was afraid to pass COVID-19 to anyone else; I wanted to be as responsible and cautious as humanly possible. I packed a bottle of germX and Clorox wipes and drove myself to CVS. Upon arrival, I advised the pharmacy technician that I had called ahead for an oximeter and that I was COVID positive. He had the oximeter waiting for me at the drive-thru window, which reminded me of the bank drawers that slide out toward the car. I made sure to sanitize my hands with the germX and wiped my debit card thoroughly with a Clorox wipe before passing it through the drawer. When the tech passed my card and oximeter with the receipt back to me, I advised that he should use hand sanitizer due to my COVID-19 status. He kindly responded that he saw me

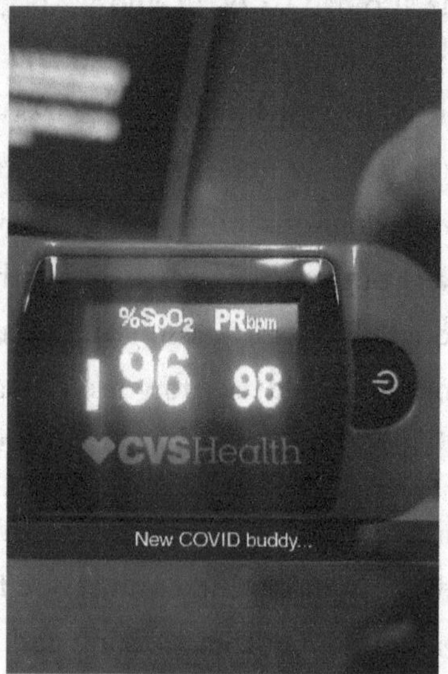

Figure 7: Oximeter – my
COVID buddy

sanitize the card and he should be good. I didn't want to get him sick or have that on my conscience, so I encouraged him to sanitize his hands, just to be extra safe. He complied with my request.

Newly supplied with an oximeter, I felt equipped enough to continue my quarantine at home, and checked my oxygen levels periodically every few hours. My dad was worried because of my compromised immune system and checked on me every day or two. It was as if I were fighting off an aggressive cold. The fatigue and pressure headaches continued and were accompanied with a heavy chest, congestion, lack of taste and smell, and a stuffy nose. I was concerned about passing the COVID virus to my puppies, but they still needed to be cared for, so they stayed with me almost the entire time since my nephew was also under quarantine. (Yes, animals can carry COVID). I managed to get up and feed them and let them out every day, a few times a day. I believe dogs sense when something is wrong, and they were extra cuddly and comforted me while I was sick and even brought me their favorite toys as gifts and laid on my side.

I reassured myself over and over, if I could just make it to the two-week mark when my quarantine ended, then my nightmare and fight would be over. I don't know why I thought it would retreat by the fourteenth day, but I had unrealistic hope. My symptoms subsided for a few days, but on Friday, October 16th, the pressure headaches returned with a vengeance and my symptoms took a turn for the worse.

My nephew battled the same cold-like symptoms, but he recovered quickly and within the quarantine period, which was expected because he was a young, healthy teenager. He almost made a full recovery, except for his lost sense of smell, and he would get winded easily when he exercised.

My symptoms persisted and grew more aggressive at the end of the two-week quarantine. I had made it to the finish line of my quarantine at home, but instead of dissipating, my symptoms grew more aggressive. I knew my compromised immune system would make my fight with COVID a tough battle, but I was unprepared for the second wave and extremely aggressive symptoms.

On the last day of quarantine, which was October 20th (my mother's birthday), I felt worse than ever and decided to go back to the doctor. The doctor listened to my lungs with a stethoscope and took my temperature and advised that I had a fever and that I did not sound well at all. He took two COVID-19 test samples, a rapid test and the "PCR" lab test that would take one-to-two days. After a brief fifteen-minute wait, the rapid COVID test results were negative for COVID-19. The doctor was convinced that I still had active COVID-19 based on his assessment of my lungs and overall deteriorating health. He instructed me to go to the hospital emergency room (ER) right away, and called ahead to notify them of my condition and to prepare them for my arrival. I returned home and asked my nephew to drive me to the ER. I did not pack a bag or a toothbrush or anything besides my phone charger because I thought I would be given medicine and be able to go home. I did not say goodbye to my puppies because I did not know how long I would be gone and did not want them to get COVID-19.

My nephew witnessed, for the first time, the severity of my compromised immune system as we battled the same illness. Mine kept progressing so much that it became urgent. I had always warned him that I couldn't be around sick people and that a cold or illness for me can be ten times worse than for others. He had never witnessed me get severely sick because I had always been very cautious about germs and avoiding people with illness. It scared him to watch me deteriorate and have to go to the hospital. He also thought that I would just go get treated with medicine and come home.

My nephew drove me to the nearest emergency room and dropped me off. I didn't want him to wait or come in with me because I didn't know how long I would be and did not want to expose him to more illness. The hospital wasn't far from our house, maybe a five-minute drive with traffic. When I arrived at the hospital, I checked in at the ER reception desk and had to sit in the waiting area until they were ready for me. I sat as far away from everyone as possible, so I would not spread COVID-19 any further.　My wait was less than fifteen minutes, which was surprising and a relief because I felt like shit. The nurse took me to a patient room and assessed my vitals. I had a fever of 103.5 degrees, a pressure headache that caused nausea and vomiting, and they diagnosed me with pneumonia due to COVID-19. They handed me a puke bag and decided to admit me to the hospital. After another brief wait, they started me on intravenous (IV) Tylenol and Zofran (anti-nausea medication), brought me a bed with wheels, and carted me off to the COVID isolation unit and started me on three liters of oxygen per minute.

(A prime example of COVID-brain fog: while writing, I could not think of the word for "bed with wheels," I wanted to say "gurney," but I was not sure, so "bed with wheels" it is.)

My first few days in the hospital were a blur and the COVID isolation unit was lonely and scary. I had to fight this virus with no visitors or family there with me. The hospital staff was amazing and cared for me like I was their family or friend. I was afraid, but felt a little safer because I was with medical professionals who truly cared despite the risk of contracting COVID-19. Any staff that entered my room was required to wear protective gear. Their safety suits reminded me of space or hazmat suits because they were all white with a full helmet and a clear face shield with oxygen being pumped in from a concentrator backpack.

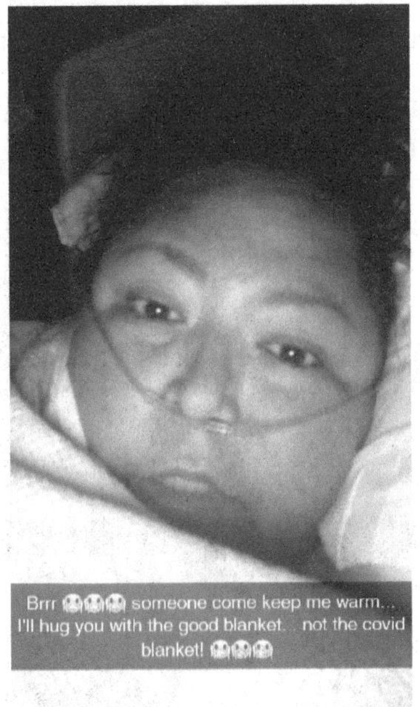

Figure 8: My first few days in the hospital

The first week or so in COVID isolation was like being at camp. I was able to get in and out of bed on my own and use the restroom and shower at will, as long as I took my oxygen tube and IV machine with me. Getting to the restroom and back to bed was difficult and tiresome. One day I sat in the hospital shower chair and let the water fall as hot as I was able to stand it for about an hour. It felt good to be able to shower on my own and that hot steam made me feel a little bit better, but my oxygen saturation levels dropped with any minimal activity.

My oxygen needs increased rapidly. I did an experiment on my oxygen dependency and was alarmed by the outcome. I took a short video where I removed my nasal cannula that was providing high flow oxygen and recorded my oxygen levels dropping on the vitals monitor. My spO2 steadily declined in seconds, from low-to-mid-nineties down to seventy-two before I put the nasal cannula back in and recovered back to above 90%. It was such a rapid, steady decline; it was almost like watching a countdown. I had one friend tell me to "Put your oxygen back on!" I didn't comprehend what was happening with my ability to breathe. The COVID-pneumonia attacked my lungs with an aggressiveness that I had never experienced with any other illness, and it was terrifying.

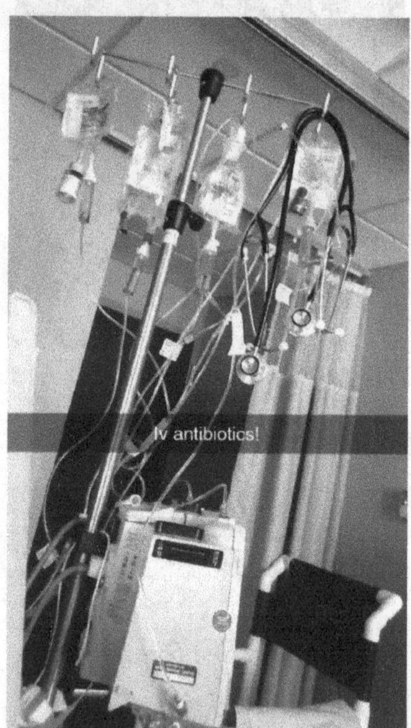

Figure 9: Finally, throwing everything at it twenty-five days after my symptoms began

COVID-19 was so new that I don't think they quite knew how to treat me at first. Since I had already been through quarantine for fourteen days, I think the medical staff thought it was too late to start the course of medication that the FDA approved for emergency use to treat COVID-19. Maybe they hoped that the virus would run its course and I would start to recover. Unfortunately, that was not the case and my health and lungs continued to worsen. I was admitted at three liters per minute, but my oxygen needs steadily increased to eighty-to-ninety liters per minute. They had to get a special machine called an AirVo that was specifically for high-flow oxygen. This nasal cannula was much larger than the small oxygen tube that went up over my ears. The larger nasal cannula had a band that went around the head to keep it in place. It wasn't until my second week in COVID isolation, starting October 30th, 2020, that the medical team decided to give me convalescent plasma, Remdesivir and everything they had to fight the coronavirus, aka Rona.

It started to get extremely scary because I was isolated with no family or friends to help me weather the storm, and the doctors began to give me an ultimatum due to my high-flow oxygen needs. They asked if I had advanced directives and asked about intubation. They were very insistent on intubation and wanted to put me on a ventilator but I said no. They told me if I did not want to go on the ventilator then I would need to sign paperwork for a "Do Not Resuscitate" (DNR) and speak with the palliative care team. I told them that I did not think we were quite there yet and that we would make those decisions when we crossed that bridge. I know they were just doing their job and had seen way more COVID-19 deaths and patients than I could ever imagine but I was not ready for either of the options that they offered. (I had previously had an unpleasant experience with a palliative care team when my mother had a hemorrhagic stroke in 2012. The palliative care representative basically wanted us to stop feeding her and let her die a slow death from pneumonia, which my brother and I did not agree with.)

After I advised the doctors and nurses that I did not want to speak to palliative care, they came anyway for a surprise visit. I calmly told them, "I know who you are, and I know what you do, and I don't wish to speak with your team, now or anytime in the future and you can turn right back around and get out of my room." I didn't yell or raise my tone; I just told them I didn't want to speak with them at any time. I felt sick, but I wasn't gasping for air, passing out, or getting dizzy and was able to function to some degree, I wasn't ready for hospice or palliative care nor a ventilator. Of all the life-threatening symptoms that I was fighting, that was the one thing that they noted in my chart as an "issue:" "Encounter with palliative care."

There were so many different doctors and nurses that came in and out of my room, it was hard to remember names or faces through all the protective gear they had to wear. While hospitalized, my medical team included internists, pulmonologists, kidney doctors, infectious disease doctors, respiratory therapists, dieticians, nurses, nurses' aides and the cleaning staff. They gave me an ultimatum: ventilator or DNR. The ultimatum was extremely scary and such a difficult life or death decision to make, especially alone, with no family or friends to help them understand my beliefs and health needs. After careful consideration, I finally told them to give me the DNR; I was going to take my chances.

The information that I had read at the time said there was a fifty-fifty chance of coming off of the ventilator for a normal person. I had zero immunity, and my odds were far less. Even if I was a normal healthy person, I would never gamble my life with a coin flip. I didn't like those odds. I decided my odds were better off being alert and without the ventilator. If that meant signing a DNR, so be it.

I knew that a lot of people were dying during that time, and I hope they knew those odds and were informed and were reading all the latest findings before making those life decisions. I think some people might have been frightened by the ultimatum and the DNR, not that that was the intention. I don't think the doctors knew what to do if I needed more oxygen than they could give me through the high-flow AirVo system. I wasn't trying to be defiant or difficult. I was just trying my best not to die and the DNR had better odds than the vent, for me, at least.

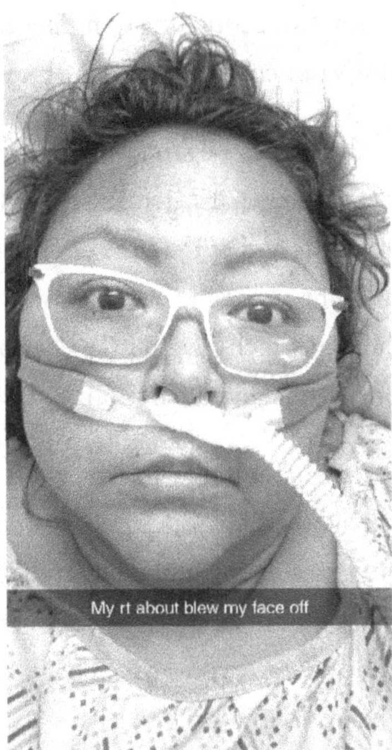

Figure 10: AirVo nasal cannula

At the beginning of November, three weeks into my hospital stay, I started to get nosebleeds due to the dry high-flow oxygen. It was during that same time that the pulmonologists recommended to start blood thinning medication due to the fact that the D-dimer was elevated and there was a high risk of getting blood clots in the lungs with COVID-Pneumonia. They added a humidifier with heat to my oxygen flow at the base connection on the wall. I declined the blood thinning medication adamantly for three or four days due to the nosebleeds and, to be honest, the anticoagulation medication scared me. I had never been on the medication; however, my grandmother was on it for years and I remember her constant bruising and bleeding that was hard to stop. I was scared that I would get a nosebleed, not be able to stop it, and bleed out.

After several discussions and reassurance from the doctors that I couldn't bleed out from a nosebleed, I agreed to take the medication, and on November 5th, they started injecting me with the maximum dose of blood thinners every eight hours. My high-flow oxygen needs increased over time to the point of eighty-to-ninety liters per minute and maxed out at ninety, I think. My "cough muscles," located in my abdomen, became sore from coughing so much. It was like I had been in a fist fight with Rona, and she punched the shit out of my abdomen.

Over the next few days, the nurses began applying four lidocaine patches to my abdomen and recommended that I get out of bed for periods of time in increments of one to two hours and at the time of feeding. It felt like my cough muscles were going to fall right out of my body. I would put my hand and apply pressure to try to hold them in which gave a little relief but not much. I was able to sit up for dinner for one to one-and-a-half hours.

On November the 8th, I remember looking at my vitals monitor, and my blood pressure was 97/37 which alarmed me. I debated pushing my call button, but I felt like the machine would be beeping with bells and whistles if I had anything to worry about. Besides, I was in the best place I could be and in great care at the hospital, especially for blood pressure concerns. That is the last thing I remember and the last that anyone heard from me.

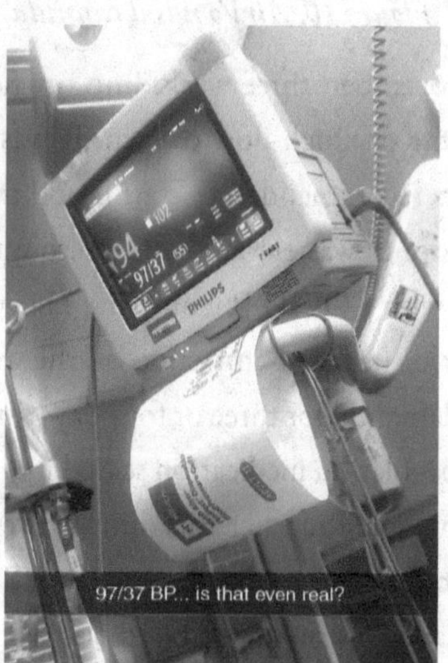

Figure 11: Vitals monitor
reading 97/37

CHAPTER SIX

BP IS THAT REAL?

In the COVID isolation unit, I was confined to my room from October 20th, 2020 to November 8th, 2020. I managed to keep in touch with my best friend, my nephew, my dad and my family daily through social media or text messages. I do not think anyone knew what happened to me or knew how close to dying I actually was, not even me. My best friend was alarmed because I stopped responding to her messages. She got in touch with my nephew and asked him to contact my dad and let him know that it was imperative to find out what was going on with me because she was concerned that she had not heard from me.

My last memory was when I took that picture of my blood pressure on the health monitor when it was 97/37. I captioned it "97/37 BP...is that even real?" and posted it to Snapchat. Everything from there went dark. Evidently, I took another photo on my phone of my vitals monitor blood pressure at 60/42. I am still trying to piece together the events that took place next.

I have gathered the hospital notes and various other resources, and I still get overwhelmed reading about it, let alone having lived through it. Evidently, I developed acute hypotension due to a hematoma and subsequent hypovolemic shock which resulted in acute injury to the kidneys. In layman's terms, my blood pressure bottomed out to the point where I went into shock.

They sent me to the cardiac ICU, hemorrhage. The internal hemorrhage was located where my cough muscles were and I blame the

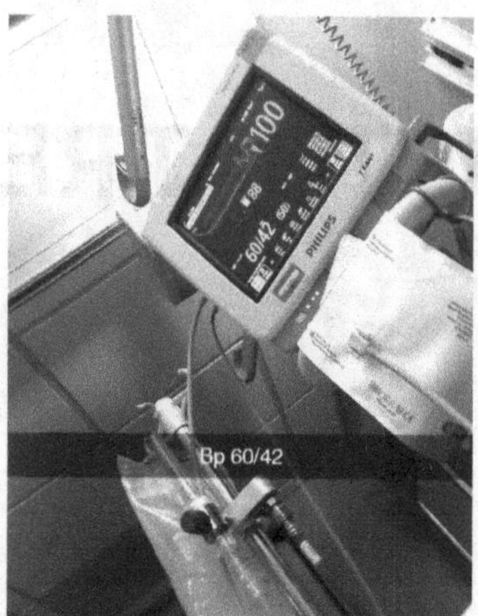

Figure 12: Vitals monitor
reading 60/42

blood thinners. The hypovolemic shock caused my kidneys to shut down and my blood pressure to drop.

They called my emergency contacts (my aunt and my dad) to make life decisions for me. The nurse called my dad and told him that I was sedated because I kept hyperventilating. They told him that they tried everything and didn't know what else to do. They also told him I was talking crazy at first, like I was not with it, and he tried to call my phone but couldn't get ahold of me. He said they scared the hell out of him. My dad, stepmom and youngest brother came to Lincoln immediately, which was a 3.5-hour drive. They picked up my nephew from my house and then they all came to the hospital. Everything was on lockdown during that time due to the COVID pandemic and they only allowed my dad to come into the hospital to see me. I had given him the authority to make health decisions for me long before the shit hit the fan. The rest of my family had to wait in the car.

When my dad arrived, the lung and the kidney doctors consulted with him right away. The lung doctor told him that if my lungs were too scarred, they would have to do a lung transplant. The kidney doctor told my dad that he had only a half-hour to decide if they wanted to try dialysis or not. My dad asked the kidney doctor if it was a life commitment and they told him, "No, we intend it to be temporary and not permanent, but there is some risk that it will not work." He also asked if they had tried the antibodies, and the doctors told him "Yes, we tried everything, Remdesivir and convalescent plasma a while ago". He asked why they didn't try dialysis on everyone with kidneys that stop working, and the doctor advised "because everyone is different." The kidney doctor informed my dad that the risks of me not having dialysis were cardiac damage or arrest, stroke and possibly death. My dad is a man of few words, but he gave them permission to start dialysis. He said, "We will try it-we have to try something."

Unbeknownst to me, I was seen by a surgeon and considered for emergency surgery. The internal bleeding caused acute injury to my kidneys. They decided to go a conservative route, stopped the anticoagulation medication immediately and gave me blood transfusions. I have no recollection of being in the ICU, having a CT scan, or of anything else that took place during that time. I was sedated because I kept hyperventilating and going into panic attacks. They kept me sedated until they transferred me out of the ICU and placed me under the direction of the nephrology doctor.

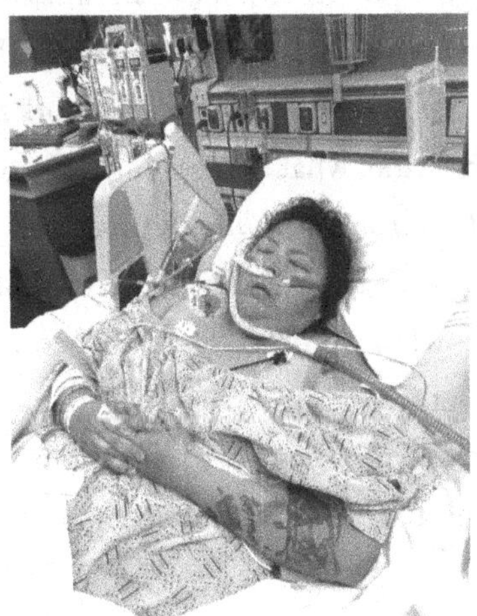

Figure 13: Sedated in ICU

I have had a few conversations with my dad about my experience after I read the medical notes and discussed writing this book. I surmised that my blood pressure plummeted to the point that set off the bells and whistles. It is unknown to me if I actually coded or had to be resuscitated, but I think they would have noted a significant event like that in my chart or in the summaries that they sent to my primary care doctor. The severe hypotension (drop in blood pressure) caused me to be unresponsive and severely injured my kidneys to the point that they shut down. It's noted that they had to give me a saline bolus overnight on November 9th, 2020 to keep my blood pressure up. That didn't work, and the following morning my blood pressure was still unstable and very low. I must have set all the bells and whistles off and I was extremely close to death. Had they not given me the saline, I believe that I would have died that night.

I told my dad that I had witnessed that exact same scenario in 2012. My mother's BP plummeted and set off the alarms after her neurosurgery from her stroke, just as my BP had plummeted. My brother wasn't there with me to make those life decisions for our mom, and I told them to do all they could for her, to at least give my brother time to get to the hospital. They gave my mom a saline bolus, which I think basically helps keep your blood pressure up to keep you alive and buys time. While my mom was fighting for her life, it was then that I felt the most alone and scared. While waiting for my brother to arrive, I realized that I was never alone. I had my higher power with me at all times: the loved ones that lived in my heart and others who walked beside me on earth. I remembered that, one time, I had filled out an icebreaker questionnaire at work and it had asked, "If you were stranded on a desert island, what is one thing that you would need?" I wrote my reply: "*Give me one friend or one family member and, together, we can survive anything.*" While at my mom's bedside praying, I remembered what I wrote and started to repeat the following words that have gotten me through some of my darkest times since: "Together, we are strong! Together, we shall overcome!" My mom survived that hypovolemia due to the saline bolus and allowed my brother time to return to the hospital. Had they not given her the saline bolus, I believe she may have died that day.

My internal hemorrhage caused hypotension (low blood pressure) and when you lose up to 30 or 40% of your body's blood supply rapidly, you start to get dizzy, tired, faint and go into shock. I went into hypovolemic shock that caused severe, acute injury to my kidneys, which caused them to stop working and to stop producing urine. When I mentioned that I had survived COVID with complications of hypovolemic shock to another doctor recently, the look of amazement on his face told me that I needed to do more research on what that meant.

I used "doctor" Google, as most people do nowadays and according to WebMD, there are four stages of Hypovolemic Shock:

Stage 1: Loss of 15% total blood volume or 750 centimeters (cc). Blood vessels constrict to try and keep your blood pressure up. Heart rate and urine are normal.

Stage 2: Loss of 750cc to 1500cc of blood. Heart rate rises. Body pulls blood from limbs and intestines to send blood to your vital organs like the brain and the heart. Blood pressure and urine are normal. Might feel some anxiety.

Stage 3: Loss of 1500cc to 2000cc of blood. (Approximately a half-gallon) Blood pressure drops. Body stops making urine or as much urine. Limbs become cold and clammy due to not enough blood. May feel confused and flustered.

Stage 4: Loss of more than 2000cc of blood. More than 40% of total blood volume. Heart races. Blood pressure is extremely low. Body stops making urine.

Hypovolemic shock can have complications such as infection, damage to kidneys and other organs or death.

Well damn, I had all of the above. There are notes from the hospital staff from November 10th, 2020 to November 13th, 2020 saying that they were asking me questions and I answered them. Sometimes I did not answer them at all, or could not, because I was unresponsive. Then there were times that I was incoherent and talked but did not make any sense. The notes sounded as if I was basically in and out of it and going through all the stages of hypovolemic shock, according to my research on WebMD.

The medical notes summarized that they transferred me to the ICU due to my low blood pressure and the critical care needs. They sent me for a CT scan with some contrast, in the area where I told them my cough muscles hurt; I have no memory of that, but that is how they found the hemorrhage. A general surgeon assessed me for emergency surgery, but said it would be a difficult surgery. He recommended stopping the blood thinners and ordered blood transfusions to try to let the body stop the bleeding on its own and replace the blood I had lost. I received eight units of packed Red Blood Cells (RBCs) and two units of Fresh Frozen Plasma (FFP). I had gained sixty-four pounds of fluid weight and was not producing urine; when I did produce urine, it was pink with blood or amber in color. My kidneys had stopped working and dialysis was one of my last options. Evidently, they inserted a central line in my jugular vein and noted that I gave verbal consent. I am glad I don't remember that at all and must have really been out of it to give consent because the jugular sounded risky. I had a catheter for multiple days and I am glad I don't remember that either. They kept me in the ICU, sedated, for several days until the hemorrhage stopped and my blood pressure stabilized.

When I first contracted COVID-19 at the beginning of October, I was able to keep in contact with my supervisor via text or virtually through MS Teams. I tried to work for the first few days because I thought the symptoms would remain mild, but the pressure headaches blinded me and I was unable to keep my eyes open. I notified my supervisor that I had COVID-19 and was under quarantine for fourteen days. It was difficult to remain in constant communication with anyone because of the arduous fight my body was enduring. None of us would have guessed that COVID-19 would become life-threatening and change my life forever.

During my hospitalization, my employer had reached out to my emergency contacts and found out that I was hospitalized. PayPal had an advocacy group and assigned me an employee advocate named Mark. I received a voicemail from Mark, who also reached out to my dad. He kept up to date on my status while I was in the hospital through communication with my dad. The company provided lodging for my family to come to Lincoln and visit me while I was in the hospital. In all my experience in corporate America, I had never had a company that provided the services that went above and beyond like PayPal did during my COVID-19 battle. My advocate made sure that I understood that I would be on short-term disability while I was in the hospital and then transition to long-term disability, if needed. I still received some compensation-I received about 60% of my income while on disability.

All of those benefits I signed up for when I first entered corporate America twenty years ago and wasn't sure what they were for? Well, this was it. Although the company provided many of the basic short-term and long-term disability benefits, I had the opportunity to add on additional insurance.

St. David's Episcopal Church in Lincoln had me on their weekly prayer list. I had many members of St. David's reach out to me or send me cards and flowers. I attended St. David's occasionally and I am very grateful for their compassion, generosity, and prayers.

While I was hospitalized, my friends, Joan and Stephanie, set up a GoFundMe account to help my family with medical or other expenses. If you are not familiar with GoFundMe, it gives people the opportunity to read a short story about your situation and then they can click a link to donate to the cause. The money is then held in an account that was able to be transferred directly to my bank account. The service provided cost a small nominal fee. Thanks to all the generous donors, they raised over $6,000.

CHAPTER SEVEN

OUT OF THE SHADOWS

My eyes were open, and I was talking, but I didn't know where I was or where they were taking me. I was being pushed on a gurney and the gentleman nurse at the helm advised me that I was still in the hospital; he was transporting me to a new room, but it was still a part of the hospital. I didn't recognize the place, and everything was confusing. I was scared of not knowing my destination and where I had come from. We entered a small, dimly-lit room that had a sink and small area with a window and blinds. I asserted that this was not the hospital and I demanded to know where we were. The nurse advised that this was my new hospital room on whatever floor it was. For argument's sake, I asserted again, "This is not a hospital, where am I? This room is too small and that isn't even a bathroom" (as I pointed at the small closet looking door.) In my mind, all hospital rooms had a bathroom. I thought, "Maybe I am dreaming; am I dreaming?" My dad was there, and he reassured me that I was still in the hospital. The nurse told me that the door I pointed to was a bathroom; he opened the small, closet-like door and what do you know, it was a bathroom. It felt like I was in a dream and I was still not convinced that I was in the hospital. Having just lost my last argument, I decided to remain quiet and just observe and plan my escape. My mind was racing and my anxiety was off the charts. When did my dad get here? Too many unanswered questions and the uneasy feeling of not knowing where I was wiped me out. I did feel safer that my dad was there with me, so I decided to rest and sleep.

I don't think that I slept long because my dad was still there watching TV when I woke up, in the tiniest hospital room I had seen yet. When I woke up, I didn't say anything; I was still observing my surroundings. I noticed they had a hospital dry erase board which had my name, "Danielle," on it, and 1500 cc h20 in the restriction section, along with my dad and my Aunt Meredith's phone numbers written on it. If I remember correctly, my dad was watching sports or something. I felt groggy so I didn't really pay attention, but I felt ill at ease in that room.

I remember laying there half-listening to the television, which was on a really low volume setting. My dad must've been trying not to wake me. When I looked around the room there were large shadows flying above me. They were different sizes and shapes, and the shadows gave me an uneasy feeling that I didn't like. I had seen the dark shadows before, and I'd always believed shadows were a dark energy. In fact, the last time I had seen dark shadows was two or three summers prior, when I was in Las Vegas. That summer I had had my own room and didn't bunk or split rooms with anyone. The bathroom door was a wood frame with a large glass insert that was frosted and dark shadows passed by the closed door a few times. I prayed on it and they either went away, or I was too drunk for the rest of my trip to notice them again.

My dad realized that I was awake and began to talk to me, asking if I was okay. I know I acknowledged him but I don't quite remember what we talked about. I remember that my voice was extremely weak and soft from being in isolation for so long, but I managed to ask,

"Dad, do you see the shadows?"

He replied, "What shadows?"

I said, "The ones flying around the room."

He said, "Do you mean the floaties you get in the eyes?"

I said, "No, I know what the squiggly floaties are, but no, not the floaties, the actual dark shadows flying around the room."

He responded, "No".

I said, "Ask Baby Trooper, he will know what I'm talking about."

Unbeknownst to me, I had just woken up from an induced sedated state (coma) and my kidneys didn't work. I think my dad thought I was still out of it. He didn't stay too much longer after that. I asked him to bring me my confirmation cross that I had received when I was confirmed at Our Most Merciful Savior Episcopal Church as a teenager in Santee, Nebraska. I considered myself a devout Dakota Christian; my cross and the power of prayer had gotten me and my relatives through some very dark times, and I wanted it to help me through these uncertain times with the shadows circling me. I told my dad that my cross was hanging on my shoe rack, and he should see it when he entered the front door to my house. We said good night; he kissed my forehead before he left and promised to be back the next day.

My cousin, Baby Trooper, is my dad's nephew and my first cousin. He was well into his sobriety journey and on the Red Road, *C'anku Duta*[3]. He is knowledgeable about our traditional ways, and I knew he would know of the shadows that I talked about.

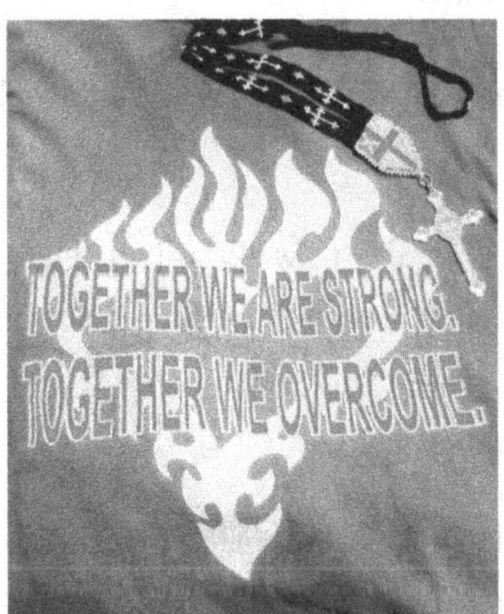

Figure 14: Confirmation cross

The next day, my dad came back, and he was so happy to see me awake and alert. He had remembered my cross and found a place to hang it. I asked him if he was able to reach Baby Trooper and he said no. I am not sure if I scared him or if he didn't want to know about the shadows, or both, so I never brought it up again. We had a good visit that day. I was finally fully coherent and understood that I was still in the hospital, but I still wasn't clear on exactly what had happened in the previous days that led up to me being taken to the room I would refer to as the "shadow room."

My dad started to fill me in on little pieces of what had happened when he had arrived. He advised that my eyes were jaundiced, and he could tell that I was "out of it". He said I was being rude to the hospital staff and wanted to go home. Apparently, when I realized he had arrived, I looked at him, had a complete 180-degree change in attitude and was as nice and happy as could be, saying in a drunk-like, excited, happy slur "Hi Dad!" I had no idea that I lost my ability to walk due to atrophy from being sedated for several days. He said I was trying to check myself out of the hospital and wanted to go home. This is how he described how I found out I lost my ability to walk:

The hospital staff told me, "You can't go home, how are you going to get there?"

I replied matter-of-factly, "I will walk home."

They said, "You can't walk."

I asked, with defiance and with disbelief, "Who can't walk?!? I can't walk?!?" and pointed toward myself.

They affirmed that I was not able to walk, so I tried to get up and walk to prove them wrong, but was unable to stand or even get out of bed. My dad said I just sat there in a silent pout, stewing in my defeat and frustration with not being able to walk and being proven wrong.

My also let me know that I was transferred out of cardiac ICU to the kidney department, and they were preparing to start me on dialysis because my kidneys had stopped working. The shadow room was the place I was waiting for dialysis.

In my upbringing, I thought that dialysis was a lifetime commitment and that I would need dialysis for the rest of my life, and that sparked fear for the impact on my future. When the kidney doctor came in to check on me, my dad did most of the talking. He asked what the plan was and how I was doing overall. The doctor explained that the internal hemorrhage had caused acute injury to my kidneys, and they had shut down. The doctor stated that the plan was to restrict fluids to get the fluid weight off and to start dialysis in order to kickstart my kidneys to try and get them to work, and then we would go from there. When we asked if I would need dialysis for the rest of my life, he advised that if this process was successful, I would be able to stop dialysis in a few days or once my kidneys started to function on their own again. I felt relieved that there was hope that I would only need dialysis temporarily and that it would not be a lifelong commitment.

I wasn't fully aware that I had an internal hemorrhage, or of all the trauma that I had experienced. I didn't know that I had put on over sixty-four pounds of fluid in a matter of days or that I had been sedated for several days, and that the doctors had considered putting me on the ventilator. Thankfully, my dad knew that I didn't want to be on the ventilator, so that never happened. Thank God that I never signed the DNR and kept putting it off by saying we would cross that bridge when we got there. No one could have predicted I would hemorrhage internally due to the blood thinners. Had I signed that DNR, I would have surely died when I was hypotensive.

I was extremely thirsty- apparently 1500 cc is not a lot of liquid, especially after being in a coma for several days with no food or water. I drank up my portioned water within the first six hours of my first night. 1500 cc is only two hospital cups of water, which is why they have the measurements on them to track your intake; they also track how much urine you output. My nurse was in disbelief that I had drunk all my water in that short amount of time, and no matter how charming, persuasive, or *uns'ica*[4] I tried to be, they would not give me more than 1500 cc of water. Since I drank my limit, they only allowed me to have little sips of water from those miniature dixie cups to take with my pills. That was a pretty tough lesson to learn on the first two nights on liquid restriction.

On the second full day in the shadow room, they had a special team come in to insert a central line to prepare me for dialysis. The lady that arrived was older; she was a super nice *kuns'i*[5] and she visited with me during the entire procedure. She performed the procedure with remarkable precision and I could tell she had been doing her job for years. She had an amazing bedside manner and she wished me well. Once the central line was set, we were able to start dialysis. The dialysis machine looked antiquated, like a huge supercomputer or something from the '80s. I guess I had never seen a dialysis machine before, but I had given plasma before, and I was expecting a smaller machine, similar to the IV machines or plasma-separating machine, instead of the big boxy machine that I was hooked to.

My dad hung my confirmation cross on a nail right by the entrance to my hospital door. I still felt uneasy, like I was being watched. I felt that the shadows were still close by, either outside or around. Even though I was on the fifth or sixth floor, I had my nurses close my hospital blinds every night when it got dark because I did not like the "eebie jeebies" that I felt while I was in the shadow room.

I found out that I could have little sodas, so I asked for a Diet Sprite. They gave me an 8oz can of Diet Sprite with ice in a Styrofoam cup. They subtracted the 8oz Sprite from my 1500 cc of water, dang it! Another liquid lesson learned; my restriction was not just water; it was all liquid. I did not know that I had retained so much fluid because my kidneys had stopped working. I had convinced a couple of nurses to give me little shots of Diet Sprite after I had hit my liquids limit. They thought I had a great sense of humor and, if you don't know me personally, I can be very charming, persuasive, and unrelenting in a hilarious, almost innocent manner. I am also a fantastic negotiator. One day, I debated with my doctor and got him to increase my liquid intake to 1800 cc. I know 300 extra cc does not sound like a lot, but, if you were in my predicament, that was HUGE! Plus, I received my little shots of Diet Sprite from my favorite nurses. One nurse was very strict, though; she was an experienced nurse and one of my main staff members at nighttime. She was overconfident and made me feel burdensome, so I tried to not to push my call button too much when she was on duty, and I didn't dare ask her for little shots of Diet Sprite or water.

The shadow room was dimly lit anyway and the only time the sunshine came through the window was early in the morning, but I slept so much that I had always missed it. Then, super early one morning, my nurses came in and gave me a bed bath and opened the blinds where the sunshine hit my face. I basked in the sunlight and felt a sense of calm meditation. That somehow signified that I was going to be okay and the shadows had finally left.

The dialysis worked and my kidneys started to function on their own again after a few days. They eventually stopped dialysis but kept the central line in for the time being, just in case. When the kidney doctor determined that I was stable, they transferred me to a different area of the hospital and out of the shadow room. I haven't seen any shadows since.

CHAPTER EIGHT

ATROPHIED

Thankful to be out of the shadow room and have my wits about me, I was hit with a stark new reality that I was unable to function on my own, or even get out of bed due to atrophy. I was confined to my hospital bed and 100% dependent on the hospital staff for everything. I don't remember how I felt when I found out I could not walk or stand, other than what my dad told me-which is kind of funny in hindsight, considering the way I worded things and tried to prove the doctors wrong because I didn't know that I could not walk. "Who can't walk? I can't walk?" in my defiant, "don't-tell-me-no," attitude and tone. The physical therapists (PT) told me that every day stuck in bed without exercise or movement takes three days of physical therapy to get back. I weighed over three-hundred pounds with untreated Rheumatoid Arthritis and oxygen dependency, and now I could no longer stand up or walk at all. My anxiety grew worse every day that I was in the hospital without getting physical therapy or exercise.

I was extremely fearful that I may never walk again because of the severity of my Rheumatoid Arthritis and not having full functionality of either knee. I had been in the hospital for over twenty-three days, oxygen-dependent and with atrophied muscles, and every day I continued to stay there tacked on another three days of physical therapy to get my muscles back-but I was still too sick to go home. After they treated all the trauma and emergent issues I had from the internal hemorrhage and hypovolemic shock, I was back to fighting COVID-pneumonia and hypoxia, but I was no longer in isolation and could have one visitor per day.

I used to be body conscious and ashamed because of my weight and would be shy or timid of showing any part of my exposed body or of being naked. Any shyness that I had previously went right out the window when I became 100% disabled and dependent on the hospital staff. My catheter was removed when I no longer required dialysis and was stabilized. "Urinary incontinence" was the new vocabulary word. No, I did not lose my ability to feel or know when I had to use the restroom. I wouldn't allow them to put adult diapers on me. I attempted to use a bedpan but that was extremely uncomfortable, and they expected me to pee and poop in that thing. I could not move or reposition myself with my own strength and when they rolled me onto it, my bottom was on the bedpan and elevated and my spine and back was lower, on the bed. I have arthritis in my lower spine, so you can just about imagine how uncomfortable and awkward that was. I was able to use the commode, but I would have to push my call light and wait for the hospital staff to come ask what I needed. If I needed to use the commode, they had to call a second person to help lift me out of bed and onto the commode. They were unable to lift me by themselves, so they used a machine lift.

'Every time I used the commode, I had to be rolled to one side as the staff put a half-folded lift pad underneath me, then rolled to the opposite side as they unfolded the pad and adjusted it until it was fully underneath me. The remote-controlled lift machine was permanently attached to rails and guides above my hospital bed and stored on the wall at the head of my bed. When the lift pad was tucked securely underneath me, they used a remote control to position the lift bar directly above me and lower it down to connect the loopholes located in the four corners of the lift pad. Once connected, they used the remote to lift me toward the ceiling with enough height to move me off of the bed and guide me into position to lower me onto the commode. I only had a hospital gown on at the time so my bottom was exposed while they dangled and swung me across the room. It reminded me of the claw machine, and I was the fluffy toy being picked up from the claw and dropped on the commode. In one instance, a male nurse walked in, looked up at me dangling high up from the lift with an exposed bottom, and he turned right around and walked out without a word. I found the look on his face and his abrupt exit mildly amusing.

I learned to have a strong bladder because there would be no quick running to the bathroom in my foreseeable future. When I had the urge to go, I pushed the call button and waited for someone to answer through the intercom and ask what I needed. Anytime I had to use the restroom, I waited for them to find another person because the lift required two people, at all times. It was the same process mostly: those two then rolled me back and forth to position the lift pad below me and then used the remote to lower the lift in position and attach the lift pad with me in it to the lift. Then they would use the remote to lift me and the rails on the ceiling to position me above the commode and use the remote to lower me on it. Most times they positioned me awkwardly and I was unable to readjust my position because I had zero leg or arm strength to lift my body weight. I secretly learned to use the lift remote, so that if they left me attached to the lift bar or it was within reach, I could reposition myself on my own using the lift machine. Most times, they disconnected me from the lift. The nurses would leave the room and let me do my business. I had to push the call button again and wait for them to come help me off the commode since I could not stand up on my own. Sometimes they would stay in the room and change the dry, square absorption pad that was underneath my bottom. They would remake my bed or change the sheets, and make sure my pillows were readjusted. I was not their only patient, so they went about other chores and sometimes it was a long, cold wait being literally stuck on the commode.

When the staff came back to assist me into bed, they would have to lift me up above the commode, high enough to wipe and clean my bottom area. I started to get bed sores on my bottom from being in the hospital bed for an extended period of time so they applied a special paste, similar to diaper cream-in fact, it might have been diaper cream. I could sense some staff were annoyed with having to lift me up out of bed every time I had to use the commode, so sometimes they used a Pure Wick. Most others were very polite and encouraged me to get out of bed at every opportunity and even started to sit me in a recliner for an hour or so each day, or as much as I could stand it, even if it was more work for them to get me in and out of bed.

There were times when I wasn't able to hold it long enough for the staff to round up a helper and go through all the motions to get me airborne and on the commode in time, so I went in the bed. The bed mishaps were few and far between, but they were unpleasant to have to be cleaned and rolled around like a burrito to redo my bedding. They no longer had to lift me out of bed so they changed the bedding and cleaned my bottom and private area and gave me a new gown while I laid in bed. They accomplished this by rolling me left and right as many times as they needed to get the job done. I didn't feel humiliated like I thought I would. My shyness was gone and I did the best I could to wait, but when it gets to be twenty-to-thirty minutes or more, it gets harder to wait and sometimes you really, really, have to go. The other bathroom tool they used was the Pure Wick system, which was a wand absorption contraption that was inserted like a catheter and it captured and soaked up the urine so I did not have to be hoisted every time, I could just go in bed and there would literally be no mess to clean up. The Pure Wick was a weird thing to get used to- it felt like you sat on pee all night and I thought it was gross-but it was better than a catheter or going in the bed. I was 100% dependent on the hospital staff, not incontinent, so in hindsight, I am unsure why they used a Pure Wick-maybe for convenience, and I rarely asked for one unless I felt burdensome to get out of bed, which was subjective to and dependent on my anxiety.

I felt utterly helpless after my near-death experience and being 100% dependent on staff for bathroom needs, water, food and grooming. This was no longer like camp, where I could get in and out of bed to potty or shower at will. This was war! A war that I was losing. I could no longer stand up on my own or even reposition myself in bed. I am still astonished at how quickly my mobility and functionality dissipated due to atrophy.

I knew that I would survive and go home eventually, but I was unsure if I would have the ability to walk. I thought that I could be confined to a wheelchair part-time or full-time. The people who determined the aids that I required to be released to my home advised that I would likely need a walk-in shower and possibly a stair lift. The stair lift cost a little over $4,000 and insurance did not cover the expense. The remodel needed to accommodate my handicap needs was going to be another expensive cost. Thankfully, my younger brother, Devin, and my dad were able to do most of the work to tear out the tub and get a walk-in shower kit. I used most of the GoFundMe funds to cover the cost of materials. It took several weeks and multiple trips for them to travel from Santee to Lincoln, which was 3.5 hours one-way, to complete the work. Thankfully, my employee advocate was able to help with the cost of hotel stays on a couple of the trips. The rest of the GoFundMe money went towards groceries for my nephew. We were so blessed with the generosity from so many people. Without the donations and help from my family, my journey home would have been delayed and maybe would have hindered my aggressive goal setting.

CHAPTER NINE

OXYGEN HUNGER

I had been in the hospital for twenty-seven days or so, and was fresh out of the kidney ward or nephrology. I am not quite sure what they called the dialysis place, but I called it the shadow room. I was apprehensive about being out of COVID isolation because I was worried about catching COVID again. The doctors assured me that I couldn't catch COVID again, but I didn't believe them because I knew that I had no immune system. I don't think that they even knew whether or not I could be reinfected because COVID was so new. It wasn't because I don't trust easily, but because I had first caught COVID in early October and was symptomatic on the 5th or 6th. The standard timeframe given to everyone at that time was to quarantine for fourteen days. I did that, but my health deteriorated. I went to the hospital on October 20th, tested positive for COVID again and was placed in the COVID isolation unit. They then said I should quarantine for twenty-one days. They tested me again on October 30th or October 31st and I was still positive for COVID. Then they changed it again and said to quarantine for up to thirty days. By this point, I was still quarantined and in isolation. They finally stopped testing me for COVID and told me that the test was invalid. They had to explain it to me about two or three more times before I reluctantly agreed to leave isolation (like I had a choice of which room I stayed in at "Chateau Hospital".)

It took a while, but my anxiety subsided and I was happy to have finally made the turn for the better. I realized that I had a long road ahead of me and I was daunted by being incapable of movement. Now that my kidneys and BP were stable, I was only being treated for COVID-pneumonia and hypoxia. The doctors started to address some of my underlying issues, such as my sleep apnea. I was on continuous high-flow oxygen, but I was down to forty liters per minute; the goal was to wean me down to five liters per minute so that I could be transferred to a skilled nursing facility. The steroids that they gave me were similar to the meds used by my rheumatologist when I had a severe flare-up. Although I had been off my arthritis medication for more than a month, I was not in excruciating arthritis pain. In normal circumstances, I wouldn't have been able to walk or move due to arthritis pain and locked joints. However, my body was so busy fighting with COVID and all the complications that I never experienced arthritis pain while in the hospital- plus I think the steroids helped. They gave me so many steroids that it spiked my blood sugar, and they had to give me insulin to regulate my blood sugar even though I was not diabetic. I could not move or walk, but that was from atrophy, not arthritis.

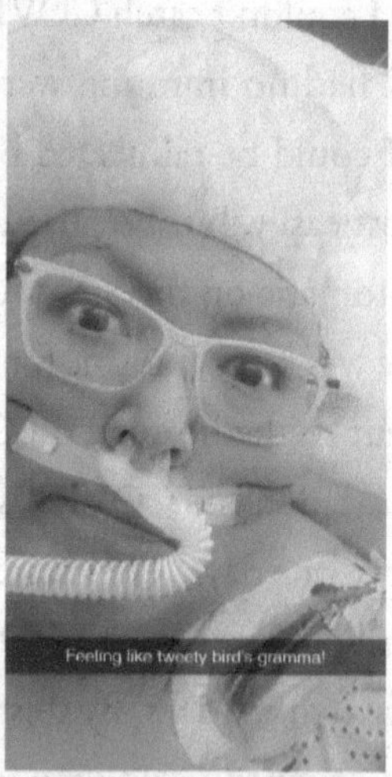

Figure 15: Bed bath
shampoo cap

My apprehension about being out of isolation subsided and I was glad to see faces and started to recognize my regular nurses and doctors. Some nursing students were there periodically as well. The University of Nebraska Medical

Center (UNMC) students wore red scrubs, and the Bryan kids wore blue scrubs. The students were trainees and were assigned to the floor or rooms, and would stop by for hourly check-ins to see if I needed anything or if I was in distress. They would be the first ones in when I pushed the call light and would help move me to the commode or the chair. They gave bed baths if it was needed. Most bed baths came from the nurses or techs. The dry shampoo hair cap felt amazing when they warmed it up, but I looked like "Tweety Bird's" grandma with that cap on. The antibacterial wipes were not always heated or lost their heat rapidly and made me chilly. There would be a tech on each side of me and they would wipe me down from shoulders to feet. They gave me a hot washcloth so I could wash my own face and neck. Plus, I received a fresh new gown and fresh bedding. They would roll me on each side to wipe down my backside.

The most memorable student visit was when the doctor asked if she could bring in some students and assess the thinning, raw skin on my bottom. I agreed-I figured *"Sure, why the hell not."* I had pretty much lost all of my shyness anyway with bed baths and beyond. It was not like I could run away if I tried. I could have said no, but figured that if getting medical attention on my bottom in front of a bunch of students would help their learning, then I was willing to do that.

The teaching doctor was very compassionate; I could tell she cared about her patients' well-being, and also wanted her students to have a good bedside manner and to pass her knowledge on to them. I got all that by the way she talked to me and asked me assessment questions or if I was okay when they rolled me on my side because it affected my oxygen levels. I was fine and told her where the sensitive parts were when she asked. I learned right along with the students-only I couldn't see my own ass on display for learning, so I just listened. She assessed that I had open wounds and prescribed a medicated special powder and paste mixture that would protect the open wounds and help them heal. She also ordered thicker absorption pads for additional cushion. Once they were finished with the assessment, they made sure I was clean, medicated and put back in a different position than when they found me. She made a point to the students that patients who were incapable of movement needed to be repositioned every two hours to help prevent open sores or infection. Once I was comfortably repositioned, they left.

The nutritionist came in almost every day to get my food preferences for the day and following morning. At first, I tried to eat what was on their regular menu, but I had no taste. It wasn't just the hospital food: *nothing* sounded or tasted good. I even ordered a hot dog and mac and cheese. I mean, you can't really mess that up. Nope, I didn't like that either. I'm old-school, so I'm used to not eating when I don't like what's served. However, the nutritionist told me that if I didn't like what they had to offer that day, I could order whatever I wanted: cheeseburgers, chicken sandwiches, fruit, pop. DING! They probably regretted letting me know that.

I ordered peanut butter and jelly (PB&J) sandwiches for lunch, with fresh fruit and a Diet Dr. Pepper. Then the nutritionist would break down how many breads, fruits, protein and vegetables I needed, so I would add in more fruit or more PB&Js. I usually did not eat very much and somehow, I found out I could order snacks, morning snacks and evening snacks! The cafeteria opened at midnight and if you had a favorite night nurse, you could have them order food for you after midnight as well.

I figured out that they rotated the breakfast entrees-usually scrambled eggs, sausage and pancakes once or twice a week. I didn't like their breakfast sausage, the eggs were bland, and the pancake was ok. My favorite breakfast became what I called "old people's breakfast" because it reminded me of my grandparents and included: two boiled eggs, toast, fresh fruit and coffee. I ordered that almost every other day. Then I would order a morning snack, which would be fresh fruit, celery and peanut butter. I didn't even know that I liked celery, but I needed a veggie in my diet. It turns out that I do like celery! Lunch would be PB&Js and fresh fruit, more fresh fruit and Diet Dr. Pepper. Evening time snacks would be PB&Js and fresh fruit. I found out that if I wasn't hungry, I could save the PB&Js in case I got hungry in the middle of the night. They had snacks and pop at the nurses' station on my floor, 24/7, and I could get cookies, milk, ice cream, crackers and soda or coffee from the nurses at any time. The nurses station only had Diet Coke, so I had to get all my Diet Dr. Peppers from the cafeteria. Not every night, but once in a while, I could get my favorite nurses to order me some PB&Js and fruit and Diet Dr. Peppers after midnight. I would save my fruit to have with my coffee in the morning, since breakfast didn't arrive until 8 AM or later and I was usually awake at 5 or 6 AM.

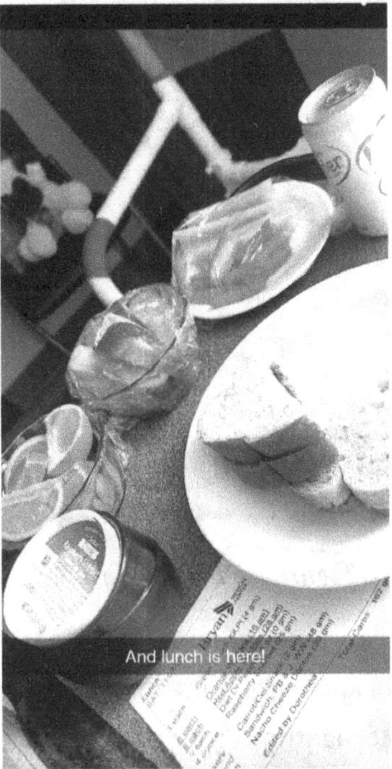

*Figure 16: PB&Js and fruit kept
me alive*

One day, I was ordering lunch and I told them I wanted a Diet Dr. Pepper, PB&J, fresh watermelon, fresh apple slices, fresh orange slices, celery, carrots and sherbet for dessert or something like that. When I was done the nutritionist tallied up my calorie count and it was low, and I was like, do I need to add something in? She said no, I had one of every food group. Then she asked about dinner, and I was like PB&J, fresh fruit, and Diet Dr. Pepper. I got a funny look, but I met all my food groups. When I received my plate, it was an array of fresh fruit, veggies and PB&Js. I did like their grilled chicken and would get that a few times a week, at lunch or dinner-never twice in one day, though. I ordered pizza once, but I didn't like that, either. I am pretty sure PB&Js, fruit, and old people's breakfast kept me alive and provided the energy I needed to start my comeback.

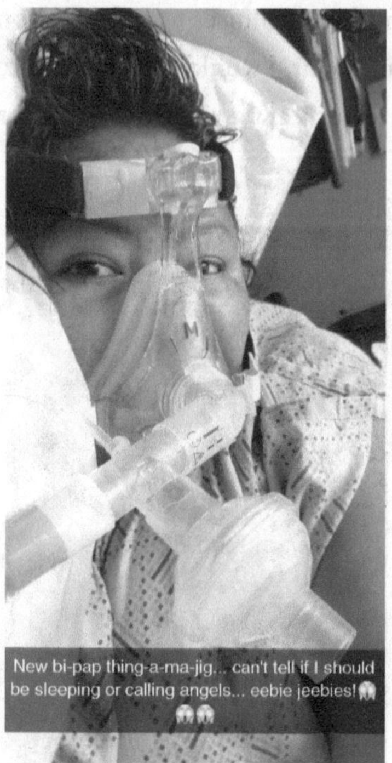

Figure 17: BiPap Machine

I had good days and bad days in the hospital. My mental health was overwhelmed by all the trauma I had experienced, my inability to do anything, and being dependent on oxygen. At nighttime, they tried to put me on a BiPAP machine which, in theory, blew air in and out while I slept. However, it was too much for me and I couldn't handle it-it felt suffocating. It is a weird feeling, having air being forced into your lungs and sucked back out on someone else's time-or maybe it was my time. But it felt like I had no control over the in-and-out timing. That, or I was having a panic attack. Next, we tried a CPAP machine, which is what I have at home, and it only pushes air in. Logically, I knew the CPAP machine provided air so that I didn't stop breathing when I slept for my sleep apnea. No big deal, I had used one before. They even hooked my oxygen tube to the CPAP machine so the oxygen flowed continuously to maintain my oxygen levels. But then something within me changed. They removed my nasal cannula and gave me a face mask for the CPAP. As I laid there trying to go to sleep with the CPAP mask on, my mind just went into panic mode. I could not breathe. I did not have enough air. My respiratory rate increased rapidly. I thought that I was going to suffocate and die. I pushed my call button. I had a full-blown panic attack the very first night I tried the CPAP and they had to take my CPAP mask off and put my nasal cannula back on. They talked me through deep breathing exercises to calm me down. I didn't know it at the time, but I was experiencing "oxygen hunger". The doctor prescribed me Xanax and melatonin to help me sleep. That first night, I stayed up until the wee hours of the morning and could not shut my mind off, even with the Xanax. It took quite a while for me to get used to sleeping with a CPAP mask again. That anxiety and panic attack was new, and it scared me because I didn't comprehend what was happening to me. It went against my logical reasoning and would impact me more later down the road.

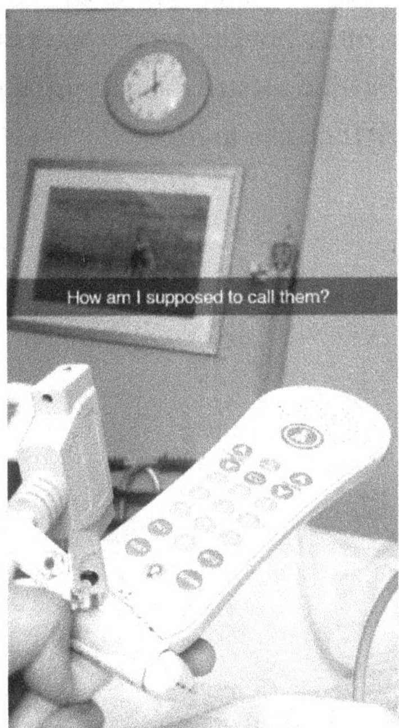

Figure 18: Unhooked call button

One night, I dropped my call button on the floor and couldn't get to it. I can't quite remember what I needed, but it was not urgent, so I decided to wait for the hourly check-in to ask for help. An hour had passed, and no one came to check on me and I think I might have had to use the commode after that long wait. I used my cell phone and googled the hospital's general number and called it. I asked the switchboard operator (Do they still call them that?) for the nurses' station on my floor, which I believe may have been level five. The operator asked me which building I was in and I told them that I had no idea which building I was in, but asked if they could look me up by name and gave them my name. After a brief pause, I was transferred to a nurses' station. I said "Hello, this is Danielle in room #xyz and I could use some help in here. I would have pushed my call button, but I dropped it and I'm unable to get to it." This wasn't the last time I had to call the operator due to a non-working or dropped call button. They told me that they would send someone in to check on me right away. After about ten minutes, I considered calling them back, when someone popped into my room and handed me my call button. I informed her that I needed to use the commode and she said she would let my nurse know. She told me that she was from a different nurses' station and then left my room. I thought that that was a stroke of genius, to use my phone to call the nurses' station because my call button wasn't within reach-but that time it was an epic FAIL! (Palm to face).

CHAPTER TEN

BLOOD THINNERS PART TWO

The lung doctors were still concerned about the high-risk of blood clots in my lungs with COVID-pneumonia. They recommended that I go back on blood thinners again, even after I had had the internal hemorrhage and almost died. I understood the risk and their concern, but I kindly declined.

It became a debate with the doctors- every, single, day. They kept trying to change my mind about the anticoagulation medication, listing out the pros and cons about the medication vs. the high-risk of getting clots in the lungs. From their viewpoint, they had witnessed plenty of COVID illness and death, and they were genuinely concerned for my safety. From my viewpoint, I wasn't trying to be difficult, I was just trying not to die. The blood thinners damn near killed me the first time and I didn't want to go through that again. I honestly did not think I would ever survive that ordeal again.

One day, my favorite primary doctor entered my room. He was one of my favorite doctors because he took the time to listen to my opinion and take it into consideration. He never talked to me in doctor-speak and he always made sure that I understood my health issues. He had a way of explaining things to me in a mutual language we could both understand. He could tell that I was adept at knowing when something was not working with my body, and that I trusted my instincts above all else. On this particular day, I could sense that something was amiss, and he had a look of defeat about him. He came in and assessed me by looking at my vitals and listening to my lungs. He mentioned the blood thinners. Doctors rarely sat down to talk to me, but he pulled up the doctor's stool and sat down next to my bed so he was at eye level. He explained the risk of blood clots in great detail. He advised that if a clot formed in the lungs, there was not much time to catch it. They could do a special surgery and insert an umbrella-like mesh thing to catch the clot before it traveled to the heart or the brain. The surgery he described as an alternative to blood thinners, but it came with extreme risk, and there was no guarantee that they would catch the clot in time. If they were unable to catch the clot before it went to the heart or the lungs, then they may not be able to save me, and I would surely die. He paused for a moment before he continued. That is when I saw the genuine sadness in his face, eyes and mannerisms. He had been on the frontline of COVID-19 and witnessed its adverse impact on people and had witnessed things I was unable to fathom. He began again and told me, "I had a patient, not unlike you, but a little older. My patient was finally making a turn for the better." He continued, "The patient was alert and responsive. He was awake and talking to me, just yesterday." He took another pause before he proceeded, then continued by saying, "Today, just this morning, he died. He was brain-dead. And I do not want to lose you or another patient like you."

We sat there in silence, as I reflected on the glimpse of the sorrowful loss of his patient. If I could have moved or functioned, I would have offered to give him a hug, because I felt like he really needed one. The loss of life-of losing patients-was giving him a sense of defeat and helplessness from being on the frontlines of the COVID pandemic. I also didn't want to die or for him to lose me too. Upon careful consideration, I told him that I would give the blood thinners another try with a caveat-that they only gave me the absolute minimum dosage. He agreed. He let me know that the plan going forward was to continue to treat my pneumonia and the blood thinners would reduce my risk of clots in the lungs. He informed me that he wanted to try to wean me off of oxygen, or reduce my dependency to a maximum of five liters per minute, so that I could be released. Then I would be able to go to rehab to work on getting my muscle and mobility back. I had never had a doctor sit down and talk to me with so much genuineness and I felt moved by what he shared with me.

I had deep sympathy for his patient that had died that day. I almost died and I was alone, in isolation. I was familiar with being frightened and the uncertainty of what was to come next, as a COVID patient. I couldn't imagine the experience that the doctors and nurses were navigating with the new COVID-19 virus and being in uncharted territory. I had been in isolation all this time and had no idea what was happening outside my hospital room, other than what I saw on TV.

That was my first glimpse into the reality of what the doctors and nurses were going through and how much of a toll the fight against COVID-19 was having on them. I felt compassion for the doctors, nurses and other COVID-19 patients, as everyone's experience was unique-there wasn't one fix-all remedy because the coronavirus was so new, and treatment was exploratory and not guaranteed to work.

I don't remember if it was that day or another day, but I cried a lot towards the end of my hospital stay. I was an emotional mess dealing with my situation and all the trauma I had experienced. The lunch person brought in my lunch, which was mashed potatoes and ham, I think. I remembered when they left, I started to eat my lunch but then began to cry, reflecting on my own experience and what the doctor had shared with me. My dad was checking on me daily and when he asked what I was doing via text, I told him that I was crying in my mashed potatoes.

It was a crapshoot whether people with the coronavirus would be asymptomatic or have symptoms that were mild to severe, or fatal. Some people had contracted the COVID-19 virus and never even knew they had it; either they had no symptoms, or their symptoms were mild enough that they never thought it was COVID-19. That made it very difficult to contain the virus and it spread like wildfire.

The exploratory, emergency-use medication, coupled with known treatments for symptoms such as blood thinners, Mucinex, steroids and antibiotics was the best-known remedy that we had at the time. It definitely was a trial-and-error time because everyone reacted differently to various symptoms and treatments. According to the Centers for Disease Control (CDC), there were 350,831 deaths in the United States from COVID in 2020 alone.

There was a minor waiting period to get the blood thinning medication from the pharmacy, but I was in no hurry as I was very reluctant to take the medication to begin with. When the nurse arrived with the medication, I began to ask how much of a dose they were giving me. In hindsight, I am not sure how I knew that they gave me the maximum dosage of blood thinners when I had my internal bleed, but I did.

When the nurse stated the amount that I was prescribed, I asked her to explain to me what the maximum dose was and how the dosage was calculated. She advised that the dosing was weight-based and that I was receiving 7500 units. I asked what the maximum was, and she said 10,000 units. In my mathematical brain, I wanted more clarification and asked, "So just to be clear, I was prescribed 75% of the maximum dosage?" She replied, "Yes, because it is based on weight". I informed her that when I spoke to the doctor, I only agreed to take the anticoagulation medication because it was going to be the absolute minimum dose. She stated again that this was the minimum dose based on my weight. I explained that I knew that I was overweight, and I understood what weight-based meant. However, I didn't agree to receive 75% of the maximum dosage. I refused the medication because I was aware that they couldn't give me medication or treat me without my consent. I asked if the doctor could reduce the dosage amount? I could tell that she wasn't used to anyone ever challenging or questioning a prescribed medication amount based on weight, or at all, really. She was a bit flustered when she left.

She came back and let me know that the pharmacist was going to call me in a few minutes to explain it to me. She found my hospital phone and unwrapped the cord around it and made sure it worked and set it on my bedside hospital-tray table. I don't think I had ever used the hospital phone because it was never plugged in, or too far from my bed, or I didn't know where it was. I thanked her and, sure enough, the pharmacist called almost immediately and explained to me what weight-based dosing was. I was steadfast in my logical reasoning and still didn't agree with it. I declined the medication again and let the nurse know when she came back to check on how the conversation went. Eventually, she was able to get a doctor to talk to me and they explained the weight-based dosing amount to me also. I declined the medication a third time.

I finally realized that none of these people understood the mathematical logic that made me unwilling to take the anticoagulation medication. I had to change my approach and needed to ask them the right question for them to consider my point of view. I then asked the doctor, "Hypothetically, if I was not overweight, and weighed one-hundred-fifty pounds, what dose would you administer then?" After careful consideration and a review of the medication on the computer, they replied "2500 or 5000 units" (I cannot quite remember which.) I finally agreed by saying, "There, that is the amount that you can give me-the absolute minimum dose. I do not care one bit about the weight-based theory; I think 75% of the maximum dose is way too much, especially because it caused complications and I don't want to have another hemorrhage."

After I landed on an agreeable dose, they started to give me heparin every eight hours through injection with a needle. When the nurse arrived with the medication, I was alert and needed to verify that the amount that was being given was what I had agreed to. From that point forward, every eight hours, I asked them what medication they were injecting me with, asked them what dose amount they were administering, and then asked them to show me. I wrote down the time and amounts that were given on a little brochure someone gave me. This regimen continued until I was discharged.

One night, a nurse came in one hour early to administer my heparin because she had a lunch break, was ahead on her rounds or had something going on at the scheduled eight-hour injection time. I declined the medication and insisted that the minimum dose couldn't be given until eight hours had passed; I didn't want an overlap in medication by an hour. In simpler terms, I probably should've just told her that it terrified me. I could tell she was annoyed by my astute concern for my well-being and medication regimen. I stayed awake that night and waited for the eighth hour to pass, because she would be back to wake me up again anyway. The eighth hour passed, then the ninth hour passed, which was fine because I did not like that medication anyway and I was hoping that she had forgotten. I was not that lucky. She came closer to 9.5 hours after my last dose. I wrote the new time down on the timeline chart that I kept on my brochure. I was now off by more than an hour than the usual time. I wasn't trying to be a pain in the ass, but I had just been through the worst experience of my life due to blood thinning medication, and I was scared of it. I wasn't about to turn a blind eye and not know what amount of anticoagulation medication I was being given, like before.

CHAPTER ELEVEN

WAITING FOR DISCHARGE

I was able to have visitors-only one per day-but I had little to no energy so I didn't mind. My dad visited me every day until I was stable from dialysis and my life was no longer in danger. They eventually had to go home for work and school. My nephew came to see me a few times. I was so happy to see him; I had happy tears of joy the first time and tried not to cry every time he visited. I had made it-I was alive! I half-jokingly told him to bring the puppies by sneaking them in, but I knew they would cry for me if they had to leave.

My nephew had to grow up extremely fast during that time. Neither one of us could have predicted that I would be gone for such a long period of time. This was the first time that he was on his own for a prolonged period. He was only eighteen when we got COVID. During my hospital stay, he was home alone and continued with his college courses, took care of our puppies, budgeted and cooked and cleaned for himself. I was so thankful that I had taught him how to meal plan, cook and save leftovers before the pandemic happened. I sent a couple of my friends over to help clean the house and help with some of the laundry. I felt that for a young person his age to be inundated with so much responsibility while in college was overwhelming. I was concerned with his grades and with his ability to focus on school. My friends helped with household chores to lessen his burden, and their help was extremely appreciated.

My nephew told me that, when Grandpa came and my health declined to the point of critical, he had had a panic attack. His heart raced and it felt like he couldn't breathe and he almost hyperventilated. He was able to calm himself down, but he said it was scary and he was worried about me. I told him that it was a very scary time. When the hospital calls family in, it's usually not a good thing. The only really happy thing that happens at hospitals is babies and he can't have any of those until after college and he gets married. I told him that during that time of crisis, I would've had a panic attack too and sometimes it can be a normal reaction to stress, worry and trauma. I asked him if he wanted me to set up any counseling or wanted to talk to someone about it. He didn't think he needed counseling. I told him if he ever needed to talk to someone and it was not me, or if I was unavailable, he could always call Grandpa or his dad.

When we discussed my COVID experience, he didn't know the full story of what had happened to me when they called my dad down to Lincoln. He did recall that they wanted to put me on a ventilator and that I had to do dialysis. I explained to him that I was well-informed about COVID before we caught it. The literature at that time gave the odds of 50% chance of coming off of the ventilator or dying, which is basically a coin flip. I told him that I was relieved that my dad knew that I wouldn't want to be intubated, which means they sedate you and have the ventilator breathe for you while you try to recover. I didn't like those odds because, with my lack of a working immune system, my odds would be much lower.

I had always let my nephew know that I had little-to-no immune system due to my arthritis, but he had never seen me sick before. I explained that, because of my condition, I am a germaphobe and hypochondriac and I try to avoid illness and sick people at all times. That was the first time I had been that sick since he came to live with me, and it was scary to see how fast and far it took me down. He was surprised when he found out that I was diagnosed with arthritis at such a young age and how severe it was.

The thought of me never coming home had never crossed his mind. He is an optimist, like me, and doesn't think the worst. The experience of having to live alone while I was in the hospital for over a month showed him that he wasn't prepared to be out on his own. He was also happy that I had taught him how to meal plan and cook before I got COVID. I didn't sugarcoat it-I told him that I had to go to another facility after they let me leave the hospital and relearn how to walk. My goal was to get home by Christmas. It was such an aggressive, almost unrealistic goal since Thanksgiving was coming up within the next week or two.

You should've seen the bruises all over my body from being on blood thinners. My bruised skin was literally purple. I had large bruises on my back, sides, arms, everywhere. It was so bad that my bestie brought me coffee and breakfast one morning, and she asked if I knew I was bruised so badly. I really didn't but I could tell she was concerned, and she wanted me to have my family look at the bruises. I could see the ones on my arms, and

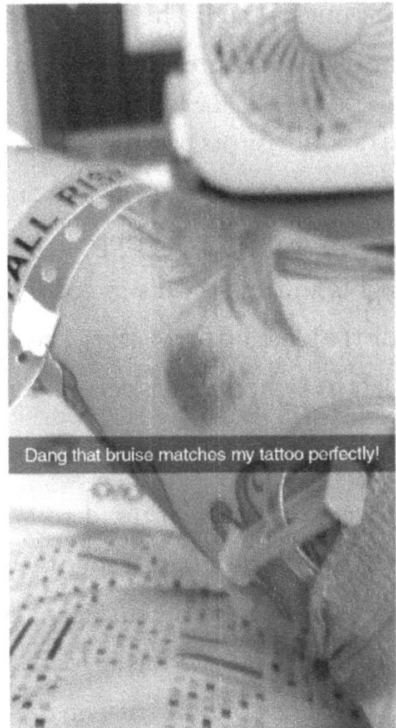

Figure 19: Deep bruises

they were so purple they matched my tattoo, which has a deep purple in the fancy shawl dancer. The nurses noticed and remarked about the severity of my bruises. I would tease them and say they threw me down the stairs and kicked me around a bit. I mean, they could have-I had no memory of about five to seven days. I knew that they didn't though, and I was not as concerned about the bruises. I figured the rest of my body was that purple color, and I remembered my grandma's extreme bruising from any little bump or hard touch, which was one of the reasons that I was scared of blood thinners to begin with.

I only had four visitors during my time at the hospital. The hospital had a very restrictive visitation policy, only one person per day. If my bestie came in the morning, she would be my one visitor for the entire day. I don't remember if she could have left and come back or not. My dad was there during my critical care time. My nephew came to visit a few times. My younger brother Devin came to see me once when he and my dad were working on my house. My best friend was my most frequent visitor and we played Yahtzee a few times.

Sometimes my hospital phone would ring, but either I could never get to it in time or never knew where it was until it rang. They still use landlines with cords, so it was usually hanging in the blood pressure cuff basket, on the floor or unplugged.

I was a little self-conscious about visitors because I was scared of being exposed to COVID-19 again. Plus, I couldn't taste or smell, and did not know if they could smell the commode next to my bed. I was so happy to see them once they arrived, however, that those thoughts and anxiety dissipated quickly. Besides, it was not like I could get up and tidy the place up for visitors. I could barely push myself up if I slumped over to the left or right or fell asleep sitting up, so they put pillows around me like a fort.

My oxygen needs improved, and they wanted to wean me off the AirVo, high-flow oxygen machine, so they could use it for other COVID patients. I was apprehensive at first about going back on the smaller nasal cannula because of my anxiety. After I thought about it, though, I was all for it, and anxious to get out of the hospital sooner than later. They put me back on the small nasal cannula that came directly from the hospital oxygen system through the wall connection. I had been there for more than twenty-five days by this time. I told them that if I passed thirty days, I was going to change my address and be a squatter legally by then, and they would never get rid of me (jokingly of course.) I was pleasantly surprised that the smaller nasal cannula helped with my anxiety and panic attacks-mainly because I put my CPAP facemask over the smaller tube even. Even though that wasn't the proper way to do it, it made me feel better, so I slept better.

I was extremely anxious to get out of the hospital and go to a long-term care facility to get started on physical therapy. I needed to get out of there and start the process to relearn how to walk and stand again. I was restless and hated feeling like I was withering away. I was getting some physical therapy in the hospital, about thirty minutes or so twice a week, but not consistently. I couldn't lift either leg, or slide them left, right, or off the bed any longer. I couldn't pull myself up. I could not believe how weak I was. The PT harped that every day in a hospital required three days of physical therapy to regain the lost strength and functionality. *"Great! I'm going to be in physical therapy forever,"* I thought to myself.

The hospital was ready to discharge me around November 21, 2020, but my insurance company declined my request to transfer to Bryan West's Acute Rehabilitation facility. Bryan had a bed available and they were willing to take me as a patient. However, I didn't meet the "oxygen need" requirements, according to the health insurance company. The insurance company said that I needed to have been intubated or on a ventilator. I didn't quite understand that reason because I still had high-flow oxygen needs and was up to ninety liters per minute or more. At the time of their denial, I was still on about thirty to thirty-five liters per minute of oxygen. I filed an appeal and had the hospital appeal on my behalf, which meant more time stuck in the hospital. We lost the appeal.

The case worker who was working on my discharge plan told me that she could send a request out to multiple agencies and gave me a list. I selected Madonna Rehabilitation, which was right up the street from my house. We found out that they were on lockdown due to COVID-19 and not accepting any new patients. The Ambassador was also near my house, but I declined to even apply there because that is where my mom died, and I refused to go there. I finally told them to send me out to Omaha and extend their search parameters. They found a skilled nursing facility in Ashland that had to order a special bed for me and would accept me as a patient as soon as they received the special bed. I was excited that they had found a rehab place for me to go and to get out of the hospital. I just had to wait for them to find a bed.

In the meantime, we continued to reduce my oxygen needs. I continued physical and occupational therapy whenever they offered it. Sometimes, they would skip me for the day if I was asleep or if a doctor was consulting. I started to do bed exercises on my own, but it was tough. I had no strength and could not slide my leg from side to side or bend my knee up to lift and slide my foot back towards me. I used resistance bands and worked on some of my arm muscles which were equally weak.

Every day that I was stuck in the hospital and waiting to go to rehab, my mental state took a toll. I felt like I was withering away, and I just wanted to get home to my family. I had good days and bad days. I am so blessed and thankful to have quit drinking alcohol a month or so before this all happened because I needed that mental clarity and strong mind to advocate for myself and survive this war with COVID-19. I knew that I needed to move mountains to get home by Christmas, but I was more than ready to start with Day One. I just needed to get there, and I grew more restless each day. I had received no updates from the new skilled nursing facility, and we were waiting for their approval to move me whenever they received my "special bed". It didn't look promising that I would ever get out of the hospital, and I was frustrated and fearful.

The day before Thanksgiving, I had given up and accepted the fact that I would likely be stuck at the hospital over the holiday weekend. This meant that I would not hit my goal to get home by Christmas because I felt that I needed a minimum of four weeks of aggressive therapy. I cried myself to sleep that night and figured I wasn't going home until after the 1st of the year. I missed my little family, my *tiwah'e*[6]. If my puppy Wrigley was with me, he would have puppy-kissed my tears away until I stopped crying and laid on my side and brought me his favorite toy. I just wanted to go home. I was overwhelmed-I was over being in the hospital and over being helpless. Everything was out of my hands and up to the insurance and skilled nursing place.

I sent my nephew to my dad's house for Thanksgiving that year so he would be with family and not home alone. I checked in with him via text and he was good, so I was good. He took our puppies, who were inside dogs. My dad had an outside dog named Zeus, who was a large breed dog. My nephew said when he took Wrigley (17lbs) and Fenway (6lbs) to meet Zeus, Wrigley started fake-crying and got scared-he was trying to climb up my nephew's leg like a tree. So, my nephew had to pick him up and carry him because he was fake-crying. My puppies might be a little spoiled, but Wrigley thinks he's human and suffers from "fear of missing out" (FOMO). If we made fun of his fake-diva-cry, he would get mad and paw at us or scratch at us.

I woke up Thanksgiving Day and was thankful to be alive, even if I was sad about not being discharged. Then the call came that they had received my bed and they were able to move me to the new place that very day. It never dawned on me that it was a holiday weekend. One of my nurses said it was a Thanksgiving miracle and I would finally be getting out of the hospital!

Thank God! I had been there for thirty-seven days! The nurses gave me a quick bed bath and dressed me in the comfy clothes I had brought. They had me sign my discharge papers and then we waited for my chariot, AKA, my ambulance transport. An EMT team arrived and loaded me onto their gurney with portable oxygen, wheeled me out of the hospital and loaded me into an ambulance that would take me to start my new journey to relearn to walk, meaning I was that much closer to getting home. I was so thrilled to be finally leaving the hospital.

CHAPTER TWELVE

SKILLED NURSING FACILITY

The ambulance ride from the hospital in Lincoln to the skilled nursing facility in Ashland was only twenty-seven to thirty miles and uneventful. It felt like a long ride but only because it was bumpy and loud. I was happy to be close to home in case I was able to have visitors. The EMTs who drove me over and delivered me to my destination were very nice and we had minimal conversation on the ride over. I enjoyed the quiet and the thoughts of the opportunity to start my journey to get back to my family. I was feeling very optimistic.

It took about thirty to thirty-five minutes to drive to the skilled nursing facility in Ashland. The room I was wheeled into was dark and shabby. The EMTs helped transfer me to my new bed and packed up their gurney and medical equipment. They had to get paperwork signed and, before they left, they wished me well.

My bed was remote-controlled, as most hospital beds are, so I was sitting up because it was mid-afternoon when I arrived and still light out. I was observing my new room and surroundings and thought I had traveled backwards in time. The bed that the facility was waiting for might have arrived from the '80s. It was brown in color with what looked like old lunchroom table-tops for headboards. The bedding also looked like it came from the '80s and they had these quilted bed pads-not the Quilted Northern paper bed pads-actual quilted rectangles made from cloth that could be washed and reused. I thought my sense of smell was gone, but it definitely smelled like a nursing home, which I was familiar with because I had visited my mom when she was in the nursing home. It is a very unique smell that is hard to describe. It was almost like a mixture of antibacterial wipes, soiled diapers and cleaning solvents.

The room had two beds: my bed, which was a larger bed for my size, probably a full-sized bed. Then there was the twin bed that may have been here since the '80s. It was the exact same style as my bed, old and flat headboards that looked like old plastic table-tops, similar to the desks I had in school, or the lunch tables at school. (I cannot think of the word I am looking for). The smaller bed was against the wall with the window. The window was decorated with Thanksgiving-themed decorations. The walls were dull and drab. The sliding-door closet was closest to my bed. I had a night stand with two drawers. They had an oxygen concentrator in front of my closet. A tall five or six drawer dresser that had clean bedding on top of it. The carpet was commercial carpet, thin and brown in color. There were stains in the carpet. There was a curtain partition in the middle of the room between my side and the other bed.

Thankfully, there was no one else in my room with me, but they made it a point that I was aware that they "double up" people in this facility and it was possible for me to get a roommate at any time. There were two other dressers and two older TVs. My TV did not work so I was able to "borrow" the TV designated for the smaller bed which the previous lady left and donated her TV and dresser to the facility. I wondered where she went-I figured she may have died, so I never asked. I also wondered, if I was to get a roommate who would determine which TV we would watch.

The facility was on lockdown, so no visitors were allowed. My friend Becky drove out to Ashland and delivered underwear, clothing and snacks to the front office the day I had arrived. The staff informed me that if I had money, I could make a list of things I needed to buy, as they sent someone to the dollar store once a week on Wednesdays.

The staff inventoried my items and then took everything to the office so that they were documented and labeled. They wrote my name, "Red Owl," on a label and hot-ironed the label on every piece of clothing that I had brought with me. They also changed me out of my clothes and into a hospital gown. They asked if I wore a "brief" and I was not quite sure that I understood the question. I guessed it meant an adult diaper and I declined. They seemed surprised that I was able to know when I needed to use the restroom. They brought in a commode and set it between my bed and the other bed, not against the wall but towards the wall, the same side as the bed's headboard.

I was tucked in after all the paperwork I needed to sign to receive treatment was completed. I met the director, who told me to let him know if I had any questions or issues, as his office was right next to me-but that was just a nicety.

They brought me a Thanksgiving Day meal from the kitchen, which was not hot, but a little warm. I was hungry and ate most of it, even though I still couldn't taste. I figured my days of ordering snacks, fruit and PB&Js were over. This place was super small compared to the hospital and I guessed that I had to eat what was provided, or not at all. They fed me one more meal that evening, but I don't remember what it was.

I pushed my call button, which looked like a baby monitor speaker with a little red light that would stay lit once it was pushed. When someone arrived, I let them know that I needed to use the restroom. They left for a short period of time and came back wheeling in a machine lift that was battery operated. The bottom of the lift looked like a floor pallet jack, but then there was a hydraulic lift system at the top that would only go up so far, almost like a bulldozer scoop arm. There was a removable battery and a corded remote control. They used the lift sling that the EMTs had left with me. Once the lift was positioned above me, they attached the hooks to the four corners of my lift sling. Oftentimes, they lowered my bed as low as it could go because the lift was limited on how high it could go. They used the corded remote control to lift me up off the bed. Then, while I was in the air, they would push and pull each side of the lift so the wheels would turn and wheel me backwards, then push to swing me around with my bottom toward the commode. Then they positioned me over the commode and, using the remote again, lowered me onto the commode. Once they placed me on the commode, they left the room, and I was able to have some privacy. I sat on the commode that was between my bed and the other bed, and I thought how awkward it would be if there was a person sitting or lying in the other bed. *Please, do not let me get a roommate.* I had to push my call button again and they would come help me off the commode using the same technique as when they put me on it. Similar to the hospital, when they lifted me off the commode with the machine, they cleaned my bottom and private area and applied diaper rash cream because my bottom was still sore from being in a hospital bed for an extended period of time. This facility did not use wipes like the hospital-they used toilet paper and wet wash rags. The staff emptied the commode in the toilet and flushed it and sometimes I could hear them rinsing it or spraying it out with water. Sometimes they inserted a liner in it and sometimes they did not. They threw the dirty wash rags into a dirty laundry bag or a liner bag and took the soiled laundry with them. Most staff carried the bucket with the liner into the bathroom to empty it, but, one time, a person took the liner out of the bucket and carried it across the room, and it had a hole and leaked. They put towels down and said someone would be in to clean the floor, but that never happened. There was a urine stain or streak leading from the commode toward the bathroom. I was disgusted but I didn't know who to ask to fix it since we were in isolation.

The day after Thanksgiving, a young staff member came to get me out of bed with the lift and placed me into a wheeled contraption and asked if I was ready for a bath. "Absolutely!" I was ready for a bath and so thrilled to have the opportunity. I hadn't had a bath in so long-my hair was matted, and I was ready to shave my head. I was used to being in the hospital where every room had a shower and toilet and sink area. I had not showered on my own since that first week or two in the hospital, which was late-October, maybe. While in the hospital, I got used to getting bed baths, which was a wipe down with antibacterial wipes and a dry shampoo shower cap. My room at Ashland also had its own bathroom and shower, but I didn't see it or enter it until the end of my stay. The young worker who came to get me for the bath covered me with a sheet and wheeled me down to the tub and shower room, which was all the way down the hall and past the nurses' station. It seemed really far for someone who couldn't walk. Plus having to wheel around a three-hundred-pound person in a hospital gown was no easy task for the petite person at the wheel. We arrived at the "Bath House," which was a humid room with a sink to wash hands and clean. In the far, left corner was a standup shower and curtain and a walk-in shower that could be accessed by wheelchair. In the middle of the room, there was one of those walk-in bathtubs that has a door that opens and closes. I had seen one before on a TV commercial targeting an elderly market. I thought to myself, *"How am I going to get in that bathtub?"*

The chair that I was in seemed to be made for the tub: they parked me next to it and the chair slid into the tub. It was able to set me inside the tub without much effort. My right foot got stuck on the bottom of the bathtub door. I didn't have the strength to lift my foot, so I had to use my arms to help lift my leg up and then slide it inside the tub. The door was shut when I was undressed and inside the tub and warm water filled the tub. I was so weak that I was unable to situate myself in the tub using my legs or arms. There was a large water tank contraption that the water came from-I figured it was a commercial water heater. The nurse turned on the jet streams and allowed me to sit for a while like in a hot tub. I didn't know I was supposed to bring my own shampoo and soap, so she let me use someone else's who had left or donated it. She gave me a clean washcloth and poured some body wash on it for me. I was able to wash myself with the rag but could not reach my feet or back. That first bath felt amazing! I wasn't able to dunk my head because it was only a sit-upright positioned tub. They washed my hair using a shower head spray attachment. I felt so refreshed after that bath-I couldn't remember the last time I had had an actual bath or shower. The only downfall about the walk-in tub is that I had to wait for the water to drain before they got me out. Thankfully, they also sprayed the sides to rinse the soap off and washed my legs and feet while we waited and used warm water. The nurse dried me off and helped me get dressed. Then they wrapped me up and wheeled me back to my room.

That same morning, after they put me back in bed, I waited until mid-morning before I pushed my call button and asked what time meals took place. I found out that I missed breakfast because I was in the bath. They were able to round me up some cold toast and juice. The rest of the weekend, I didn't get any physical therapy or baths. One evening they forgot to bring me dinner, so I had to ask again for a meal and was brought something cold and unappetizing.

Monday finally arrived, and I was excited to get started with my physical therapy. I was hoping to get a bath again that morning because that was the most enjoyable part of my stay so far, but no such luck. The daily routine was meals three times a day, no snacks. This was old-school-you either ate what they gave you or not at all. They told me that I could substitute a hamburger or grilled cheese or PB&J for the meal, but I had to order them in advance. The menu for the following day would be passed out with the dinnertime meal, and I needed to fill it out and return it to the staff after dinner. I didn't get a menu that first week or two, so I was not aware of the process until later. I just figured it was "eat or don't eat" for my first few weeks, which wasn't terrible because I was trying to get my taste buds back anyway.

Sometime during the mid-morning, two ladies in scrubs and face shields entered my room and introduced themselves as Janet, who was a physical therapist (PT), and Michelle, who was an occupational therapist (OT). They showed me a gait belt, and both worked to lift me up to stand. Oh, my goodness-I couldn't remember the last time I stood up and my legs felt like jelly, but I was happy that they stood me up and I wasn't in bed. I don't think I stood long because I was so weak, so they sat me on the edge of the bed. I had to lock both elbows straight to hold myself up, like a baby giraffe, so I didn't tip over left or right. They showed me some bed exercises to work on during my alone time. They worked with me for thirty minutes of combined discipline because it took two of them to lift me with the belt. When our time was up, they told me that they would be back the following day for thirty minutes and would continue to work with me for thirty minutes per day until I was able to regain some functionality to stand up and walk on my own.

Immediately, I was like "wait a minute." I let them know that the therapy plan they described didn't work for me. I wasn't trying to be there forever. If possible, I wanted a full hour of therapy from each of them and I wanted to be home by Christmas. I might have said, "I need each of you to kick my ass for one hour per day-that's two hours of therapy every day." They had to have thought I was batshit crazy by how weak I was. They gave me reasons why they weren't able to extend my time and included Nebraska state guidelines or regulations. After a brief consideration of their denial, I concluded that, "This is not the place for me; I'm not trying to be here forever. I have aggressive goals; I want to be home by Christmas and thirty minutes per day just isn't going to get me there. Can I please speak to the director or the administrator to transfer me to a facility that can handle my needs and goals?" Michelle and Janet were very nice, and I liked them right away, but thirty minutes of combined therapy per day was too low of a goal and that didn't sit well with my unbound determination to get home. I didn't hear back from anyone that day regarding wanting to transfer to another facility, and it wasn't like I could get up and go check.

The following day, Tuesday, December 1, 2020, a lady that I hadn't met came in and introduced herself as the Director of Therapy, and we had a long visit about what my needs and goals were. I wanted to know what state regulation I would be breaking by wanting longer therapy and what the exact threshold was. I wanted to see it in writing, because I wanted to know if I was wasting my time being transferred if I was just going to run into the same resistance to aggressive therapy elsewhere, but I didn't mention that to her. She advised that there was nothing in my way of getting more therapy-they just didn't want me to overdo it, and to protect me so I didn't get hurt. She said that they had no problem increasing my therapy to one hour per discipline, but that they needed to overlap for fifteen minutes in between because it took two people to lift me up and help me stand and walk. We compromised: forty-five minutes of PT daily and forty-five minutes of OT daily with fifteen minutes of combined therapy. I was happy with our new therapy plan and wanted to give them a chance. Plus, changing facilities seemed like a huge pain in the ass and with everyone on lockdown due to the pandemic, it seemed difficult to be transferred again and would have delayed my therapy more.

Michelle and Janet came to my room that day and instead of combined therapy in the middle, they decided to do it at the beginning of therapy and then split it up after that. It worked for me. I was extremely weak and couldn't stand, but with the gait belt they lifted me to a standing position. Although I needed help, it felt good to stand up. I finally felt like I was headed in the right direction and made some progress.

Michelle and Janet came to my room for daily therapy between 10 AM and 12 PM and worked with me to regain strength and to practice standing from a seated position. They called them "sit-to-stands". Even though I could not stand, I had to practice engaging those muscles again by trying to stand. Part of my therapy was relearning to dress myself while laying down since I wasn't able to get up. Putting on clothes while laying down was extremely challenging for me, and Michelle and Janet had to help me. I had to shimmy, lift or roll my hips to get my bottoms up. Even putting on a shirt was a challenge because I wasn't able to pull it all the way down and not able to sit up on my own for any period of time, in the beginning. Therapy mostly occurred Monday through Friday, and on some Saturdays. The new therapy schedule exhausted me, and I did some bed exercises in my spare time. I was extremely fatigued to the point of taking naps during the day. Plus, I was in isolation 24/7 and didn't see or talk to anyone other than the hospital staff, and there was really nothing else to do. I figured out how to login to Netflix to watch movies, but I mostly did therapy or slept.

I asked for a bath every day that first week and they said it depended on the bath schedule because they only had one bath for the facility, and they rotated people. I found out quickly how lucky I was to get a bath on my second day there.

In the morning, I used my call button to have them lift me onto the commode. Talk about a bladder control workout! I thought I had a strong bladder from the hospital, but at the skilled nursing facility I had to wait for more than an hour sometimes. One evening, I had to use the commode around dinnertime, and I pushed my call button and waited more than an hour. It was closer to one hour and forty minutes, give or take. When the nurse arrived, I curiously asked why there had been such a long wait and she advised that she was busy feeding other patients who couldn't feed themselves and told me that I needed to change my bathroom schedule. I asked, "How do you change your bathroom schedule?" I did not know that that was a thing or know how. From that point forward, I started to log when it would take longer than an hour. One evening, I googled the phone number for the facility and called the nurses' station and advised them that my call button had been on for more than an hour. There was only one or two times when my bladder couldn't wait, and I went in the bed. I attempted to try to use my call button before dinnertime to try and force myself to go, but that was not always successful.

My second bath was about a week after my first bath. This time it was an older lady who came to get me and she had a hard time getting me over the door threshold-I thought she was going to tip me over. This time in the bath, I noticed she had to spray my hair off the sides of the tub and down the drain. After my bath, she applied lotion and combed my hair for me. I felt like a kid, having a caring *kuns'i* bathe and care for me. When we returned to my room, she also changed my bedding out for clean bedding. I noticed when she grabbed my pillow it was completely covered with strands of hair that had fallen out. There was not one square inch of that white pillow that was free of a hair strand or two. It was more alarming when she flipped it over, as the other side was equally covered. I wanted someone to come shave my hair off, but we were on lockdown and couldn't have visitors. Otherwise, this facility used to have a stylist come in to do hair for the residents. At first, I thought it was odd to have a stylist come here but, in my mind, this was only a temporary placement until I reached my goal to go home. It made more sense as I picked up on clues that I may have been the youngest person there, but I was not 100% sure since I never left my room and I had never received the grand tour.

I concluded that the facility was short-staffed, and I get it, we were in a pandemic, but my basic needs were not being met. It was very daunting to have to ask for basic needs for a prideful, independent person like myself. I finally complained to the manager, and she said she was going to have a talk with the lady who told me to change my bathroom schedule. She also told me that they weren't used to getting patients like me who were able to advocate and help themselves with feeding and brushing teeth or even knowing when they had to use the restroom. I also advised that no one checked on me in the mornings, and I needed someone to bring me water and a spittoon so I could brush my teeth and wash up if I wasn't able to get baths. Things did improve for a few days after I complained, but I was extremely worried about retaliation because this was a super small facility and I was literally helpless and alone. I worried for nothing-everyone was super nice and a few of the nurses apologized for the others.

There were some super nice people there: a mother-daughter duo, who were cool and my favorites. The nurse who recommended that I change my bathroom schedule turned out to be really nice and started to visit with me. I just think she may have been overwhelmed that day. I get it, everyone was overworked in that place, and we were on lockdown. It was a stressful time everywhere, so I had no hard feelings. It just sucked to be completely and utterly dependent on others for basic human needs, like water, bathroom, bathing, and eating. A lot of the staff started to talk to me after they found out I was extremely competent and then they all found out my story and why I was there. They started complimenting me on my therapy improvements and determination. I appreciated them all because, without them, I would not have been able to do the impossible things that I needed to do to get home.

Michelle and Janet came and helped me get dressed and then got me out of bed. Once they helped me stand, I was able to walk with a walker. I am not sure if "walk" was the right word, but I could lightly lift my right foot (my strong, dominant side) forward and drop it down, and then I slid my left foot to catch up and moved in a forward direction while I leaned on a walker. In therapy, I walked from one edge of the room to the other, since we were in isolation and I was not able to leave the room. I had aggressive goals and that two-hours a day of working on shuffle-walking with a walker wore me out. Over time, I started gaining strength, and was able to do bed exercises. I was able to slide my legs left and right and could barely slide my foot back toward me by bending at the knee-not far, maybe an inch or two. I could lift my legs off the bed one at a time about a half inch to an inch. It seemed like it took forever, but time went by slowly there. I had nothing to do, no visitors and I was tired all the time from therapy. Visitors were allowed to stand at your window, which I found to be odd, but for the people who called that place home, I was able to see how that could have been enlightening. One day, an elderly man with a miniature USA flag walked to my window, knocked and waved. I was startled but I waved back, and he went on to the next window.

Michelle gave me an assignment to get myself dressed and get ready for therapy by 10 AM. She gave me some cool tools to use leading up to this assignment, like a sock contraption that helped me pull my socks up and over my heels. She gave me elastic laces for my shoes. The elastic laces kept the shoes tied. The lace elastic expanded so I would not have to tie and untie my shoes ever. They also gave me a shoehorn, which I have at home for my arthritis, that helped put my shoes on, so the backs of my shoes did not fold over when I pushed my foot down into the shoe. The other tool she gave me was a little grabber contraption-I pulled a trigger that was attached to a string, and it constricted the string so it pulled the ends to grab or pick up things.

One would think getting dressed by 10 AM would be a simple task, but I had zero strength, could not stand up on my own or walk. I was finally able to move my legs back and forth from the bed exercises and all the work I did in therapy. However, getting myself dressed was an entire workout session all on its own and it completely wiped me out.

I used the grabber to get my clothes from the dresser. I used the grabber to place my underwear in a laid-out position by my feet so I could put my feet through the foot holes. Once both feet were in, I used the grabber to pull them upward until I was able to reach them. And then it was an entire bed workout to get them up into the proper position. If anyone had walked by my window and saw me flailing about without context, they probably would have thought I was possessed. Lifting the hips up, I pulled up the underwear-if they weren't on straight or up far enough, I rolled to one side, adjusted and then rolled to the other side and adjusted, and then lifted the hips up for a final adjustment. My bed didn't have bed rails, so I almost fell out of bed a time or two. Rolling back and forth and lifting my hips definitely left me short of breath and I was on three or four liters of oxygen per minute. I took a short rest and then rolled up each leg of my sweatpants and positioned them in a way where I could get a foot in the foot hole and pulled upward with the grabber, then put the other foot in and pulled up and over the legs with the grabber. Then when I was able to reach them, I lifted the hips up and pulled and rolled left and right to adjust and lifted the hips up and pulled. I did the pants first because I was only in a hospital gown during the night. I didn't even try to deal with a bra during my time there. The shirt was a little difficult because I had to sit upright on my own to take the gown off and if I was sitting on any part of it, I rocked to the left or right to get it off. I pulled the shirt up on and over. After all that, I fell back on my pillows and rested and caught my breath.

The final piece was the socks and shoes. My bed adjusted up and down horizontally. It also could raise the head or the feet. While I dressed myself, I laid the bed flat and lowered it to the lowest position; in case I fell, it would have been a short fall. After my short rest, I rolled over onto my weak side, which was my left, and positioned my feet toward the edge of the bed. Then, I was able to push myself off the bed with my right arm and prop myself up on to my left elbow and rest there. I then moved both of my feet off the bed and pushed off on my right hand and left elbow to a seated position on the edge of the bed. I did it! I sat up on my own for the very first time! I was so proud of myself, but, that first time, I was so far on the edge that I thought I was going to slide right off. I rested for a bit and after the shock and amazement wore off, I continued. I used my sock tool and stretched my sock over the tool, put my foot in and pulled the strings up so my sock was correctly placed on my foot. I repeated the process for my other foot. Then came the shoes. I used the grabber to reach and grab my shoes that were underneath my bed by my headboard and placed them at my feet in a way that I was able to get my foot in them with a shoehorn. It took three to four tries to get my shoes on. I was so proud that I got dressed by myself but, holy crap, that was a workout and a half.

Getting myself dressed took an hour or close to it. I had ten to fifteen minutes to spare before Michelle arrived, so I decided to lay down and rest. I threw myself backwards in the bed and was able to lift my legs by using my arms and pulled on the legs of my sweatpants that I just put on. I rolled back and forth until I was back in bed with my head on the pillows. As I laid there catching my breath, I noticed that my gown was still on my bed. I leaned down and grabbed it and put my arms in it and pulled it on over my t-shirt. Then I covered myself back up with the covers, shoes and all. The only thing showing was my head and the gown over my shoulders.

Michelle arrived right on time, and as she entered my room, she noticed that I was still in bed. In a raised tone of voice she said,

"Danielle, why are you still in bed? You were supposed to be dressed and ready to go!"

I said in my innocent voice, "I was so tired from yesterday's therapy, I overslept!"

In her mad-therapist-voice, she asked, "Do you need me to get you your clothes?" She walked to my dresser and opened the top drawer.

I replied, "No."

Still in a raised voice, she asked, "Well, why not?!?"

I replied, "Because I am already dressed!" I threw the covers off and started laughing.

She said, "Ooh, you little stinker, you got me good there!"

We had to relay the story to Janet because it was just such a good prank!

It must have been about the third week-my progress was going slow, and I started to doubt if I was going to makc it homc by Christmas. I had a little over two weeks to make serious progress if I had a fighting chance. Once I got myself dressed that first time, they made me dress myself every day after that. I figured out if I folded the bed up like a human taco, I was able to reach my feet. That made it easier to get dressed than using all the gadgets. We worked on sit-to-stands every single day in therapy. They used a gait belt to lift me up because I still was not able to stand on my own. Every day in therapy I grew stronger and a little more confident. I was able to walk before I could stand, and not just shuffle-walk, but actually pick my feet up and take steps. At first, I was petrified (in my Gloria Gaynor voice) that they wouldn't be able to catch me if I fell.

They would both cheerlead, "COME ON, DANIELLE! YOU CAN DO IT! PUSH! YOU GOT IT, DANIELLE!"

Then one day, I stood up with little to no help! Oh, my goodness, they were so proud of me and I was so proud of myself. They did not let up one bit, though. We repeated those drills every day! If it got easier, they lowered the seat, the bed, or put me in a wheelchair! Day after day, sit-to-stands and walking! I worked out on my own with resistance bands for arm and bed exercises. To this day, I can still hear their voices cheerleading me on, whenever I get down on myself or when I am in physical therapy.

One day, they needed to weigh me for their records and the scale was down the hall by the Bath House. They put me in a wheelchair and wheeled me and my oxygen concentrator down to the scale. It was on an incline, and they were both standing there debating on how to get me on the scale, when I simply said, "I will just walk up there." They both turned and looked at me with amazement. Then they helped me stand up and I held on to the rails of the scale and I walked up the incline. They both looked at me with pride and disbelief, "Oh my gosh, Danielle, you did it!" Then they took my weight. I did not even wait or hesitate, I got back in the wheelchair, then I took off and wheeled myself back toward my room with my arms and shuffled my legs. I couldn't go too far because I was hooked to the oxygen concentrator.

I received another bath during my third week there. It was getting down to the wire and I wanted to be home by Christmas Eve. That meant that I had to be somewhat independent by the twenty-eighth day there, the fourth week. Janet came in and told me that she didn't think it was safe for me to go home yet and that I might have to wait until after the first of the year because we had so much more work to do. It almost seemed impossible, but I told them going in, I had aggressive goals and I wanted to be home by Christmas. I asked Janet how much therapy would I really get by staying there over the holidays? I couldn't hold back my tears and I told her tearfully, "I just really want to go home." I was doing everything in my power to get home. She empathized with me and understood my point. She confirmed that there would be a lack of therapy during the upcoming weeks due to the holiday. She told me that it wasn't a hard no, but she would talk to the director and see what they could do to make it happen and we still had about ten days. She reassured me and said, "If you want to go home, you will go home."

Throughout the last ten days or so, I was able to stand up on my own from my bed in a raised position, and with my walker I could walk myself to the commode. Once the nursing staff figured out that I didn't need to be lifted, I rarely saw them anymore, mostly for meals and meds or to check my blood sugar, which was always normal. I told them I wasn't a diabetic and I didn't know why they were giving me insulin because they stopped all of the steroids that spiked my blood sugar when I left the hospital. They finally took me off the insulin.

There were tasks that I had to complete to prove that I was ready to go home. I had to stand up from a regular toilet height, which was twenty-four inches. I failed on my first few attempts at this in the bathroom that was in my room. We worked on sit-to-stands from the bed at twenty-four inches and from a wheelchair. The bed was harder to stand up from because it had no side-rails to leverage from. I had to learn to use momentum by rocking forward with my feet centered below me and pushing myself up from my thigh muscles. I had to walk up and down four steps, which we had not covered yet because we were still doing sit-to-stand exercises. I had to walk eighty feet, which for me was to the Christmas tree down the hall by the nurses' station and back (using a walker and oxygen, of course.) Janet and Michelle rolled my oxygen concentrator down the hall behind me so the oxygen tube would come with me. I was able to do it. I was winded, but I passed. My oxygen stats would drop into the seventies or eighties but I recovered quickly, sometimes in less than a minute.

I received my final bath during week four and after every bath they had to spray my hair out of the tub. I knew hair loss was a side effect of COVID and post-COVID or stress and trauma. I saw the video from Alyssa Milano where she talked about hair loss after COVID. She combed her hair and showed the strands that fell out after simply combing it. I could relate, and I was also alarmed every time I saw my hair strands go down the drain. I had to put my hair loss concern in the back of my mind because I had to get home; it was my top priority.

I was bound and determined to go home. I felt confident that I could stand from a twenty-four-inch seated position, so we attempted the toilet sit-to-stand that I had failed before and I passed! I was able to stand up from the toilet with no help. I asked my therapists, "Where are we going to get steps?" Then they took me into their "gym" where they normally do physical and occupational therapy when not in a lockdown status. They had a set of wooden porch steps that had five steps and a small platform at the top with handrails. I went up all five steps-right foot first, and pulling my left leg up. I took a short pause and repeated the process until I reached the top. I turned around and looked at the stairs, but I was afraid that if I went down forward facing, my arthritic knees would buckle as they had done so many times previously over the years with RA. So, I turned back around and went down backwards, the same way I went up, one leg at a time, strong leg first, and slowly. They graduated me from therapy that day! I was so happy! We took a picture together and they gave me a graduation t-shirt. Wow! I did it! I was super happy! I cried tears of joy that night! I was finally able to go home after sixty-five days of being away from my nephew, my puppies, my home, and fighting for my life!

I woke up on December 24th, 2020, happy for my trip home. Everything was set up for my release. Home healthcare was going to meet me at my house after the holiday and they were going to set up my oxygen at my house on December 24th. The social worker came to my room that morning and said the company they had originally set up called and backed out, saying they were overbooked and could not take me as a new client and that I couldn't go home. I said, "Are you joking? Today is the day I am supposed to leave." I was disappointed, deflated and determined to leave. All I wanted in the world was to go home.

I asked if there was another company and she said that she had some calls out, but since it was a holiday, the odds weren't likely. I asked what exactly I needed to do to leave and she advised that I needed to have oxygen set up at my home. I asked if there was another company that would provide oxygen. I said "I'm going to walk out that door today one way or another, and you can either help me or not." She said she would do her best to try to find another company and left my room.

The social worker came back and said she found a company to provide oxygen that day, but they needed $150 to set it up. I found it odd that I had to pay a fee since I had met my out-of-pocket maximum and it was the end of the year, but I just wanted to go home, so I handed her my Health Savings Account card. She left to get the oxygen delivery set up. When she returned with my card and confirmation number, she said I still couldn't leave. I asked why, when, just a few minutes ago, all I needed was oxygen and I have oxygen now. The reason she stated was that I didn't have home health care set up, which was a nurse coming to check on me, physical therapy and occupational therapy. She advised that if I left it would be considered Against Medical Advice (AMA) and insurance may not pay for my entire stay if I left under those circumstances. I asked, "So just to be clear, you are not letting me go, because I do not have home healthcare set up, which was set up but was canceled beyond my control just this morning? And if I stay here, I would only be getting six days of therapy over the holidays or the next two weeks? And the original home healthcare company was not scheduled to come see me until after January 1st to begin with?" She replied, "Yes." I said, "Okay, where do I sign?"

I made sure that she documented that I only AMA'd because the home health that was set up was canceled that morning by the company. Once the paperwork was complete, I thanked her and I was so happy to go home. I started to get dressed and ready to go. I don't know if it was all the stress of the possibility of not getting to go home but I had an upset stomach. I tried my best to get up and make it to the commode but that didn't happen. I pushed my call button, and a nurse came and helped clean me up and get me dressed. She took my soiled clothing and bedding to the laundry room. I texted my nephew to come and pick me up, which should have only been a thirty-minute drive. The staff helped pack my belongings and we waited by the entrance.

My nephew said he had arrived, but we couldn't find him. We asked him to honk, and we didn't hear any sounds. We eventually figured out that he was in the wrong town-there was another skilled nursing facility fifteen miles away with the same name. After a twenty-minute wait, he arrived, and the staff helped load my belongings into the car. They let me borrow their walker and sent me home with one of their portable oxygen tanks. I didn't receive all my clothing back, because some was in the laundry, but I had my name on everything. They told me that they would either mail my clothing to me or send it with the nurse who was coming to check on me and pick up their walker that they let me leave with. I was so ecstatic to be going home. I have not received my clothing back nor have I heard from them since.

The goals and requirements of my physical and occupational therapy were set by the way my house was set up. When you walk in my front door there are stairs to the left. I thought that there were four stairs to the first landing, then it turns ninety degrees right and goes up to the second floor with an additional twelve steps. The stair lift was straight and did not turn the corner to the main floor, so I needed to be able to climb the four stairs to get to the stair lift. If the stair lift was to include a bend for the additional steps, it would have cost an additional $2,000-$3,000 and I couldn't afford that, but I could afford to try to walk up four stairs.

It was a collective effort to help bring me home. I cannot thank my dad and my brother enough for donating their time and travel costs to come to do the hard labor to remodel my bathroom. Without the generous donations from everyone, I would not have been able to have a stair lift and walk-in shower installed. I thank all who donated to help me get home. It also helped me purchase items that insurance did not cover, such as toilet seat risers, furniture risers, handicap bars, and a shower chair.

I have always been fearless and determined, with a crazy side of humor, a you-can't-tell-me-no attitude, and have always been up for a challenge. I set a goal to relearn to stand and walk within twenty-eight days, which gave me four weeks to be home by Christmas, and once my mind was made up, there was no stopping me, no matter how big the mountain in front of me was. Regardless of if I failed or not, I was going to get up and try.

My aggressive goals, relentlessness, unbound determination and hard work paid off with the help of the best therapists I could have asked for. I was able to stand-up, walk with a walker, and climb up and down four steps, all of the things

I needed to do to navigate my house. Even if they thought I was batshit crazy at first, I hit my goal and left the nursing home on December 24th, 2020, after twenty-eight days, and I could not have done it without Michelle and Janet.

CHAPTER THIRTEEN

HOME SWEET HOME

My nephew picked me up from the nursing home in my vehicle. Once we were loaded up, we drove out of Ashland towards Lincoln. It had been sixty-five days since he first dropped me off at the emergency room-such a long time to be away from my *tiwah'e*. He was able to visit me before I left the hospital, but he wasn't able to visit while I was at the nursing home. I was so happy to see his face. I smiled ear-to-ear and told him, "I missed you so much!" I tried my best not to cry.

I left with a portable oxygen tank that the nursing home let me borrow which only had about two hours of oxygen flow. They also loaned me a walker because I was so weak and wasn't able to walk without it. I was so ready to be home. The oxygen company that I paid $150 was supposed to meet us at my house to set up my oxygen concentrator so I would have oxygen 24/7. They called while we were on the road, and I advised that we were on our way, and we would be there within fifteen to twenty minutes. I surely did not want to miss them, due to it being Christmas Eve and a long holiday weekend was upon us. When we arrived at home, my nephew got my walker out of the car and set it up for me to use. He followed me into the house with my oxygen tank. The puppies were beyond excited to see me when I walked through the door. They jumped up and wanted me to pick them up, but I had to sit down first. I walked straight to the kitchen table and sat on our tall kitchen table chairs. It was a workout to get to the kitchen and I needed a rest. I picked them up one at a time and hugged and kissed them both. Both puppies had separation anxiety while I was gone. I tried to talk to them on the phone once, but it made them and me cry more than anything.

The oxygen company arrived while I was sitting downstairs with the puppies resting. The representative was nice, and he set up my oxygen concentrator on the main floor, and showed us how to operate it and attached a fifty-foot oxygen tube to it so I could navigate throughout my house with oxygen. I didn't try to walk through my house because of all of the activity earlier in the day of having to pack and get ready to go home. I was tired. After the oxygen guy left, I decided to go upstairs to my bedroom.

I used the walker to get back to the staircase by our main entrance and I managed to get up the steps to sit down on the stair lift. My nephew taught me how to operate the remotes and the buttons on the chair and he brought my walker up behind me. The chair swiveled so it was easy to get up from. I had to use the walker again to get to my bedroom. I was surprised-my best friend had prepared my room for me! I had all new bedding and a small decorative Christmas tree was lit with all my Christmas presents around it. It was such a nice gesture that warmed my heart. After I got upstairs to rest, I wanted to shower but I was too exhausted.

My nephew went out and got us fast food for Christmas Eve dinner, and we ate in my room since I had no energy to go back down the stairs. It went against my one house-rule-no food in the bedrooms-but I figured I had to make an exception so that I did not fall. We had a nice little visit and opened our gifts. He then went to my aunt's house to visit and play games, which is part of the family tradition. I did not mind-I was tired. While he was gone, I had to use the restroom, so I used my walker and went to the restroom next to my bedroom. I was able to see my new walk-in shower for the first time. The drywall and edging were not finished, but it looked great and there was a shower chair. There was even a parallel grab bar that sat on each side of the toilet. The only thing that had not been installed yet was the handicap grab bars on the walls. I was so impressed by all of the work my dad and brother had done. I had finished going potty and wiped my bottom and was ready to get up off the toilet, but my muscles were so weak from overdoing it that day that I had nothing left. I tried and tried to lift with my arms and reposition myself. My puppies were in the bathroom with me, but they couldn't help me. I probably tried for twenty minutes, but no matter how hard I tried, my muscles were spent and I was too weak. I finally heard my nephew come home and I hollered at him through the door that I needed help. My first day home and I got a tough lesson in overdoing it. I didn't want to go back to the hospital or the nursing home, but I needed help. Not even thinking about it, I had locked the bathroom door, but it was just one of those single hole punch locks where you can pop the lock with a safety pin or nail. It took my nephew a while to get the door open and there I was stuck on the toilet with my pants down, sweating from all the attempts to stand up. I told him I was stuck and needed help getting up. He came in and we crossed arms, and he pulled me up while I pushed with what little leg muscles I had left until I was in a standing position. I told him I didn't need help with the rest and I should be able to get back into bed. I cleaned myself up, pulled my sweatpants up and washed my hands. Although I really wanted to take a hot shower, I did not have the energy and did not want to be stuck on the shower chair. I decided to get ready for bed, to rest and try again the next day. After I was done in the bathroom and brushed my teeth, I used my walker to get back to my bedroom. My bed sat high so it was easy to get off of the bed. After being stuck on the toilet and having to have my nephew rescue me, I looked up toilet seat risers online and sent him out to buy one. They were not cheap, about $45-50. I ended up buying two, one for downstairs and one for upstairs. My first night home, my puppies did not leave my side, and we slept soundly in my own bed with a puppy nestled up on each side of me, or on top of my side.

I woke up on Christmas Day and went into the bathroom to test if I could get off of the shower chair. I sat down on the shower chair in the shower, fully clothed, in case I got stuck again. It was easier to get out of than what I had gone through yesterday of being stuck on the toilet. My leg muscles were sore from all the attempts to get up to a standing position. I was extremely weak. The toilet upstairs had a toilet seat riser on it so that I would not get stuck again. Once I passed the test of getting out of the shower chair, I decided to take a long, hot shower. It had been about a week since I had had a bath. I disrobed and turned the shower on. I was looking forward to a long, hot shower. I sat in the chair, but the water was lukewarm, not hot. I turned it to the hottest temperature that it would go, but it was still only lukewarm. It got cold fast, and I had to cut my shower short. I was so blessed to have the ability to shower after only getting four baths in the last twenty-eight days at the nursing home. I didn't think anything about the lukewarm water-I just figured that my nephew had run the hot water out or had been running the dishwasher or washer.

I mostly stayed in my room that weekend and my nephew brought me meals and sat with me to eat and visit. The puppies rarely left my side. I made my way downstairs to try and let the dogs out. I was scared of falling off of the last couple of steps, but I managed to get down them on my own. I walked to the kitchen table, but had to stop and rest. My legs felt like rubber, and I ran out of breath even though I had continuous oxygen from the oxygen machine. I had another twenty-five feet to go to the patio door to let the dogs out. "I can do it," I told myself. I walked to the door and opened it for the puppies, but my legs felt like jelly, and I ran out of breath again. I leaned on the side of my couch and sat on the couch arm so I could get up when the puppies were ready to come back in. I didn't even put a leash on them because I thought if I bent over to attach the leashes, I would have surely fallen over from no breath or pure exhaustion. My older dog, Wrigley, knew how to knock on the door when he was ready to come in and the little one, Fenway, just waited with him, or if I wasn't quick enough, the little guy started barking. Wrigley knocked on the door, so I got up and went to the door to let them in. I made it back to the kitchen table and had to sit and rest. I sat there for the longest time to rest because I knew that I needed to have enough energy to get up the steps to my chair lift and the last thing I wanted to do was fall and get sent back to the hospital or nursing home. I surprised myself-I was able to get up the steps after letting the dogs out. I just needed to learn to take breaks and be smarter about my energy. I had to go up one foot at a time and do

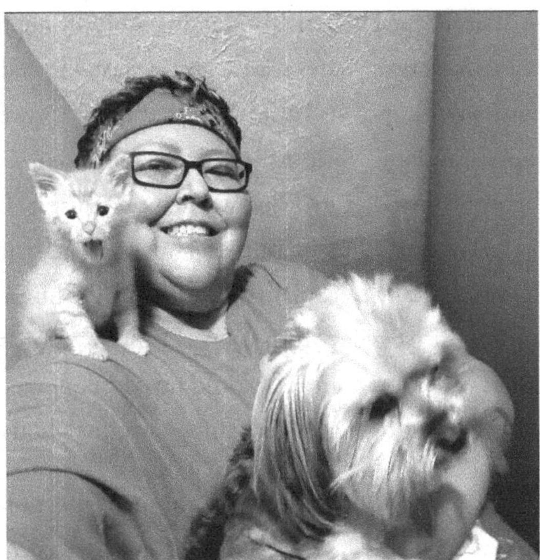

Figure 20: Stair lift rides for the pets

deep breathing to get up those steps, and my internal cheerleaders (Janet and Michelle) were cheering me on. *Come on, Danielle! You can do it! PUSH!* I made it! Fenway wanted to ride up the stair lift so I let him. And then, since Fenway went up, the next time Wrigley had to go up. And then, of course the puppies both wanted to ride with me on the stair lift every time-like it was their carnival ride. Crazy puppies! We began to foster bottle baby kittens and they would also ride up the stair lift sometimes.

I had known that I would get more of a workout being home than being stuck in the nursing home not getting any therapy, because I was unable to leave my room. At least at home, I had to get up and walk to the bathroom, and take the dogs downstairs at least once per day. My nephew had to take them out the other times so that I didn't overdo it. I was frustrated with my weakness and wanted to do things right now. I learned to be patient with myself and slow down, and took notice of my new limitations. I knew I could get downstairs at least once per day to let the dogs out and walk to the patio door. I would try to stay downstairs and sit at the kitchen table for as long as I could stand it before going back upstairs. It was quiet, and I just sat there and reflected on my journey and how far I had yet to go. I enjoyed being in my own home with my *tiwah'e.*

I was sitting downstairs at the kitchen table talking with my nephew, and I asked him if he had noticed the shower water wasn't getting hot. He said he had noticed, but hadn't thought anything of it. I told him that most showers come with a governor, or a stopper, and it likely just needed to be adjusted, since it was new. I told him he probably just needed an Allen wrench to adjust it. I tried to explain where to look and feel for the adjustment piece, but without being able to go up and show him, it was difficult to explain and difficult for him to comprehend. I had brain fog and cognitive delay from COVID and my words did not always come out in the right order, or, at times I could not think of words. In addition, he had limited knowledge of tools or fixing things around a house or car.

My nephew and I had some good visits while we spent most of the time in my room or at the kitchen table. My favorite holiday has always been New Year's Eve and New Year's Day because it marks the end to one chapter and the beginning of another. I spent that holiday at home with my puppies. My nephew went to my aunt's house to celebrate and eat Indian tacos. He brought me some *watec'a*[7].

I had a doctor's visit with my rheumatologist that first week of the New Year and asked my older brother to come stay with us and drive me there. It took me a long time to get myself ready; I had not planned for the extra time and energy it would take me to get ready and I felt like I was going to be late. I rode my stair lift down the stairs. I was able to step down, but coming off the last step, my knee gave out and I fell backwards on the stairs with my other knee bent underneath me. It wasn't a bad fall, but it was a fall. My older brother was concerned and told me that we should cancel the appointment, and I reluctantly agreed. He and my nephew helped lift me up and I sat at the kitchen table with them for a while. I knew my brother would know what I was talking about to adjust the hot water in the shower. We both agreed that there should be someplace to adjust it or to turn up the hot water heater. Then out of nowhere, like a lightbulb had gone off, my nephew said,

"Or you can get to the pipes through the hole in my wall."

Without missing a beat, I said with surprise, "What hole in your wall?!?"

He then said, "Grandpa and Uncle Devin had a leak and they cut a hole in my wall to fix it."

I asked, "How big is the hole?" He replied, "As big as my head."

That is how I found out there was a hole in my nephew's bedroom wall. My older brother was able to adjust the shower with an Allen wrench and showed my nephew what I had tried to describe to him, so we had hot water now! He didn't need to go to the access hole, the adjustment screw was located behind the water on-and-off nozzle.

Originally, my dad and I had thought that I would come home in a wheelchair and would learn how to walk from home. We had planned on knocking a hole in my closet wall to put a door there for me to access the bathroom. I texted my dad and said, "Hey, you put the bathroom door on the wrong wall-it was supposed to go to my room, not lil Beau's!" We still tease each other about it. My dad said, "Dang, Grandson told on us!"

It was about three weeks into January before the home healthcare company came to do my intake paperwork. I was so thankful that I decided to AMA on Christmas Eve, otherwise I would have been stuck in the nursing home for another three or four weeks. I was right in my hypothesis that I would get more physical therapy being in my own home than being confined to my room at the nursing home. I made it a point to go downstairs every day. I bought furniture risers to lift my couch high enough so that I was able to get up from it because it sat lower than twenty-four inches. Eventually, I worked up enough strength to go downstairs twice a day and would try to eat meals downstairs. Once my intake assessment was done, I had physical therapy and occupational therapy come to my house to do therapy with me for up to one hour, twice a week. It was hard work, and they both wore me out equally. I couldn't even lift a two-pound dumbbell when we started. I had to start with a can of soup out of the pantry to do curls and lifting exercises. I wasn't aware that I was so weak and was shocked that I couldn't lift a two-pound dumbbell-it was very eye-opening. The occupational therapist helped me do household chores like vacuuming and dishes, and we worked towards cooking a meal and regaining self-sufficiency. I couldn't do the dishes while standing-I had to pull a chair over and sit to do the dishes. I couldn't stand for more than a couple of minutes, so I was also unable to cook a meal at first.

Home healthcare physical and occupational therapy worked with me every week for about five to six weeks. We worked on sit-to-stands, general walking and balance. We worked on basic household chores, vacuuming, laundry, dishes and cooking. I was able to lift the two-pound dumbbell eventually. As the weeks went on, my legs felt less like rubber, and I was able to let the dogs out without stopping at the kitchen table for a break. I was able to cook a meal, but it took all the energy I had, and I needed to drag a chair into the kitchen to sit down. It was such a prideful feeling to be able to cook and clean on my own, even if I had to stop and take breaks or break it up to one item per day.

My physical therapist had me walk from the patio to my front door as many times as I could for five minutes-it was difficult, but it was a start to rebuilding strength. She saw my stair lift and assumed that we didn't need to do stairs because I had the lift. I told her, "Oh, no, we need to work on stairs-I don't want to use that stair lift forever. I want to be able to unplug it and not use it at all." We started at the bottom step and did one step-up, step-down with each leg five times, then ten times, and then one day I was able to walk up the steps. I may have slept for two days afterward but I was so amazed and proud of myself.

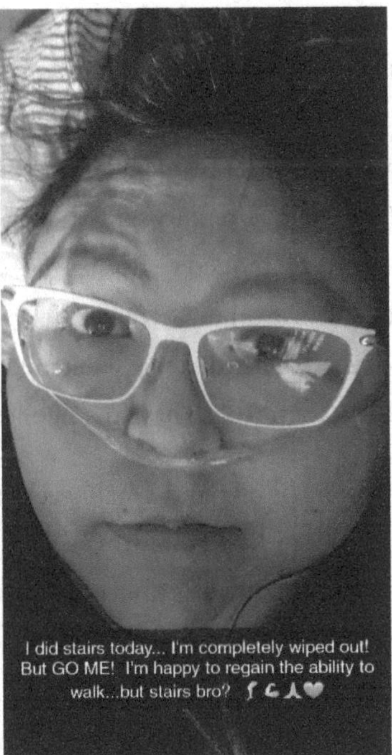

*Figure 21: After my first time
walking up the stairs*

I eventually got a new walker, plus I still had the one I had borrowed from the nursing home, so I no longer had to haul one up and down the stairs. I just kept one on each floor. I also bought a bag that held my portable oxygen tank in front of the walker so that made it easier to travel to my doctor's visits. Instead of tennis balls, I put little walker sneakers on the back walker legs to glide.

This was my new reality and it taught me to be patient with myself. It wasn't easy because I just wanted to do everything, but then I would overwork myself and was either wiped out the entire next day or risked hurting myself. One day I went downstairs, which meant I used my walker to get from my bedroom to the stair lift, seated and loaded myself onto the stair lift, and used the remote to ride the lift down the stairs and walked down the steps. Downstairs, I rarely used my walker because the hallway was narrow, and I had things to hang on to such as the kitchen table or the living room furniture or my desk. On this particular day, I walked toward the patio door, but I forgot how weak I was; I was going too fast and couldn't pick up my leg fully and it hit the carpet suddenly, which made me trip and fall. As I laid there on the floor, I was frustrated with myself for the fall, but the puppies kept me company and thought I was down there to play with them. I laid down there for some time, playing with the puppies when my nephew finally came downstairs and saw me lying on the floor. He asked, "What happened, Auntie? Did you fall?" I replied sarcastically, "Nope, I am just down here doing my exercises," and pretended to do sit-ups. As we joked, my nephew helped me up. I had a huge bruise on my left knee. It was a long learning process on how to be okay with oxygen dependency, a weakened state, and accepting that I could not do it alone. I was thankful to have my nephew with me to help me.

I fell one other time, about one or one-and-a-half weeks after my fall in my living room. I fell on the same knee. I had gone to CVS to get a prescription. The pavement directly in front of the store was uneven, so when I exited the store, my shoe caught the lip of the higher pavement and down I went on the same knee. I laid there for a minute, not sure whether to laugh or cry. A couple of concerned customers helped me to get up and took me back to my car. The manager of CVS came out and took an incident report, but I never did hear from them again. I am fortunate that I didn't break my kneecap, but my ego was bruised.

Home healthcare continued to provide in-home care until the end of February. I didn't let them know about either of my fall incidents because I sensed they would recommend that I go back to the nursing home. I then was approved to start outpatient lung therapy. I was unable to have both in-home and outpatient therapy at the same time-insurance would only pay for one or the other. I chose outpatient therapy, as I was ready to go to lung therapy to work on my lungs.

One of my therapists knew of a person that had a portable, battery-operated oxygen concentrator, so I asked if she could contact them and ask if I could buy or rent it. She was able to connect me with the person and I was able to obtain the machine. It was dusty and I could tell it had not been used for a long time. I cleaned it up and ordered new parts for it. It was not continuous oxygen, and I had to get used to using a pulse oxygen concentrator. Sometimes it didn't work at all but it was better than lugging the big oxygen tanks around all the time.

I finally went to see my rheumatologist after I rescheduled my appointment that I had canceled after my fall. We discussed restarting my arthritis medication-I was on Xeljanz right before I had caught COVID-19-but she wanted to get the pulmonologist's opinion first, and I was scheduled to see him in the next week or two. Hindsight is always 20/20-later in my journey, my rheumatologist let me know that Rituxan patients had a much higher risk of having severe COVID-19 hospitalization with manual ventilation and mortality. She stopped prescribing the medication completely. I did more research and the study published in 2021 by The Lancet Rheumatology said the increased risk ratio was between 1:7 up to 5:5, and that's when they were studying the effects of the COVID vaccinations for patients with RA that were on Rituxan. At the time, there were no vaccinations for me or others like me, or risk ratios other than the basic 50/50 that I knew of for normal people coming off of the vent. The emergency-use vaccinations were not available when I had COVID and would not get approved until December 11th, 2020, for Pfizer, and December 18th, 2020, for Moderna. They also said to wait ninety days after having COVID before getting a vaccination. The study further stated the importance for patients like me to build an immunity and recommended that immunocompromised patients be given up to three doses of the vaccine to make a difference. I was on Rituxan, also known as Rituximab, through June of 2020 and, as previously mentioned, it could take up to five years for my immune system to recover. The Rituxan wiped out my white blood cells and targeted the T-cells. I wondered how I made it out alive. I am a numbers person and I have not been so lucky at the hands I have been dealt in this life but I did know one thing-I knew survivability.

CHAPTER FOURTEEN

LUNG THERAPY

In February 2021, I was able to see my pulmonologist for the first time since I had left the hospital in November 2020. When Dr. Reichmuth walked in, he was middle-aged, handsome and very well-dressed. He was very dapper-his shoes matched his attire flawlessly-and there was a familiarity about him. I thought he had been my doctor in the hospital, but it was hard to recognize him without scrubs and a full hazmat suit. He introduced himself and confirmed that he had been my doctor in the hospital. He told me that he had been extremely worried that I wouldn't make it because of my deteriorating health and that I had been extremely sick. We went over my respiratory and breathing tests and he told me that there was some interstitial lung disease, but with COVID-19, it was hard to tell if it was scar tissue or if it was still in the healing phase. He recommended lung therapy and we agreed to start in March. I could tell that he was very happy to see me and to see that I had survived the severity of my illness and my near-death experience. I trusted him, and he would take over leading my medical team while I recovered, post-COVID. He approved the arthritis medication and I gave him authorization to communicate with all of my doctors.

At the beginning of March 2021, I met with the lung therapists at Bryan LifePointe. During intake, I was told by the respiratory therapist (RT) that it was unlikely that I would get off of oxygen. I felt deflated and defeated, but I knew that I still needed to build muscle and strength because I was still extremely weak and easily fatigued.

When I showed up for my first session of lung therapy, I was given a sweat headband that would have a spO2 monitor for the forehead tucked in underneath the band. The headband and the high average age of the group reminded me of Richard Simmons and "Sweating to the Oldies." It was easy to get used to the lung therapy ritual. We would start with stretching and resistance exercises. Then we would do ten sit-to-stands, and then we

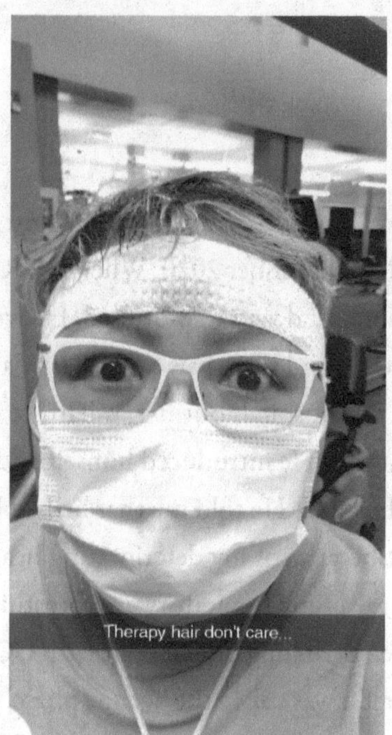

Figure 22: Lung Therapy 1

were prescribed five to ten minutes on a machine, I was assigned an arm bike and a NU-Step which was like a seated mountain climber machine. Eventually, they also added in a five-minute walk.

I grew strong enough that I was able to stop using my walkers. The lung therapy program was twelve weeks, and I just went through the motions of the class. We had educational information sessions after our workout maybe once per week. Otherwise, we would do cool down stretches. I lost my momentum on regaining my ability to walk and functionality. I attribute it to being told that my lungs would not heal, and I could not get off of oxygen by the RT who did my intake. It deflated me and I felt defeated before I even started the class.

The state of Nebraska was dolling out COVID vaccinations based on age and high-risk category. I had extremely high anxiety and was anxious to get a vaccination to give me a fighting chance, should I contract COVID again. Just about the time that vaccines were going to be available for the high-risk group, the governor kicked my group down the list and kept the priority based solely on age. I had a minor panic attack and finally called my dad to see if I could drive to my hometown to get the vaccination and he recommended contacting the Ponca Tribe, who had an IHS clinic in Omaha that was a lot closer. I called them and thankfully the Ponca Tribal Health Center was able to vaccinate my nephew, myself and my brother in March, instead of waiting until my age group would be next on the list. They had a vaccination clinic at their office in Lincoln for our second dose, so we did not have to drive to Omaha, which was very convenient. Thank you to the Ponca Tribe of Nebraska Health Centers.

It was about halfway through the twelve-week session when I decided that the RT intake person had no idea what they were talking about. COVID-19 was so new, how could he possibly know, especially if my pulmonologist, who had been on the frontline during the COVID pandemic, was optimistic about my ability to heal. I decided, "I'm not dead yet, so I'm not done yet!" From that midway point forward, I built my momentum up and started working out every day that I did not have lung therapy. I took my portable oxygen tank, which I named "Fred," to the gym that I was a member of and started to work out in the pool. I have always loved working out in the water, because it was less painful for my joints, and I had better flexibility and mobility than being on land. It was a workout session just to get ready to go to the gym. I had to pack my clothes, towel, shower supplies, aquatic shoes and resistance dumbbells and ankle weights. In addition, I had to make sure I had enough oxygen in the portable tank or change out the tank for a new tank. I had six full tanks on hand on a consistent basis. I loaded all of my bags and equipment into the car and drove to the gym. I had to unload all my stuff and take it into the gym. I wore a mask at all times, even in the pool. I had a twenty-five-foot oxygen tube that I attached to my tank and sat it beside the pool lane that I had reserved for that day. I then put my workout gear beside the tank and entered the pool at the end where the stairs were. I walked down the stairs forward facing with no issues, one step down at a time with my strong, right leg, then the left would follow. Then I took my mask, glasses and nasal

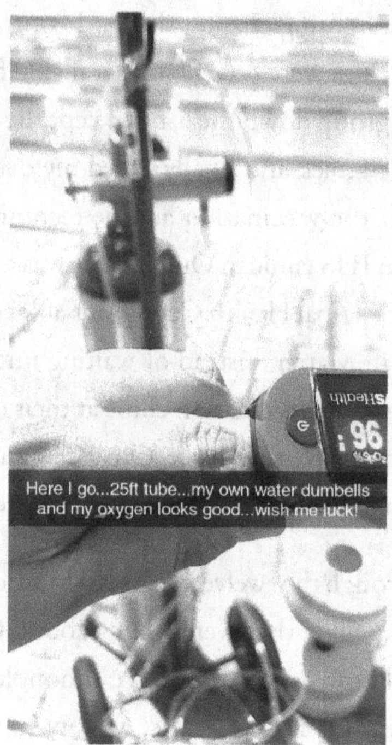

Figure 23 Aquatic Therapy

cannula off and held them above water with one hand as I dunked myself under the rope, then when I came up from under the water, I handed them over to the hand on the proper side of the rope. I repeated that process until I reached my destined pool lane. The oxygen tube only stretched to half of the length of the swim lane. I often walked laps, side-stepped and did kicks for my leg workout. Then I did arm curls, by lifting water or pushing water, and used water resistant dumbbells or ankle and wrist weights. My entire workout lasted roughly one hour with a cool down and stretch period. One time, I accidentally went too far and pulled my oxygen tank into the pool, and an elderly lady yelled at me to notice. I turned around and saw Fred in the pool, so I mildly panicked and started to tread that way, until I noticed that Fred was floating. There my oxygen tank was, upside down, with its wheels bobbing up and down like a buoy. Fred fell in the pool at least three times in total.

One day, I walked into the pool face forward, as per usual, but on that day, I had forgotten my aquatic shoes at home, so I went barefoot. On the second or third step down into the pool, my foot slipped forward and I fell into the pool and under for a full dunk. I popped up and noticed the people sitting around the edge of the pool and I said loudly, "WELL THAT'S ONE WAY TO GET INTO THE POOL!" I got zero laughs. I think the bruise to my ego from no laughter was bigger than the bruise I was going to have on my ass. The bonus part of the workout was that I would soak in the hot tub for fifteen minutes after each workout if there weren't any people in the women's hot tub located in the women's locker room.

In May of 2021, I had the confidence to travel back to my hometown for my relatives' memorial dinner. In our culture, after our loved one's pass, we typically have memorial ceremonies after one year of mourning, which was the hardest, then again at five and ten years. Through time and as our elders have passed on, it seems like the five- and ten-year memorials went with them because it is very rare that I see those anymore. I wore my mask at all times, but it was the first time I had traveled and I was gifted a motorized handicap scooter from my friend's boss. I was self-conscious about my portable oxygen machine at first, but I was so happy to see all my relatives and friends at the memorial dinner that I hardly noticed my oxygen machine. My nephew and I stayed at the *Ohíya*[8] Casino and Hotel about ten miles from Santee on Hwy 12. I invited two of my closest friends and biggest advocates, Shelly and Roberta, to meet me for breakfast at the casino before I ventured back home. I met Shelly when I was in Jr. High, and she worked briefly for my uncle's construction company in the office before she became a science teacher. She was the coolest science teacher ever! We had a unique bond right away from the beginning. She would eventually be my teacher, but we became very close friends. She is one person who has always believed in me, ever since we met. Roberta, I met later when I took classes at the Nebraska Indian Community College-she was my English professor, and we also had a unique bond. I think she really enjoyed my stories and my raw and authentic writing ability-that, and I was super funny. I always told her I wanted to ride her motorcycle. Roberta and Shelly shared an office at the college, so it was easy for me to go in, and we would get lost in stories. I think if you were to ask them their favorite story of me, it might be the time I jumped on an airplane and went to Washington, D.C. by myself, not knowing a single soul, and came back with lifelong friends.

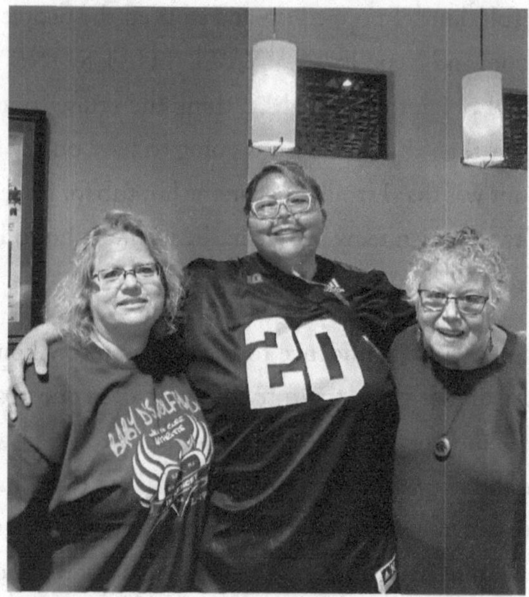

Figure 24: Shelly, Me and Roberta, May 2021

We had buffet-style breakfast with my nephew and Roberta's husband. I told them a bit of my story of what had happened to me, at least what I had known then, and both teared up and were so happy that I was alive. They teared up, so I teared up. I forget how much I have been through until I see it on other people's faces, if that makes any sense. It was so good to see them and get a hug-it had been years since I had seen them both. Roberta was retired and Shelly no longer taught in Santee. Their favorite story of mine now might be this one. I had always told Roberta that I wanted to write a book, but that was back when I was a talker, not a doer. I know that if you have at least one person who believes in you, you can do anything. My motto became; "Together, we are strong. Together, we shall overcome!" I am lucky enough to have both of these strong women to have believed in me since we met.

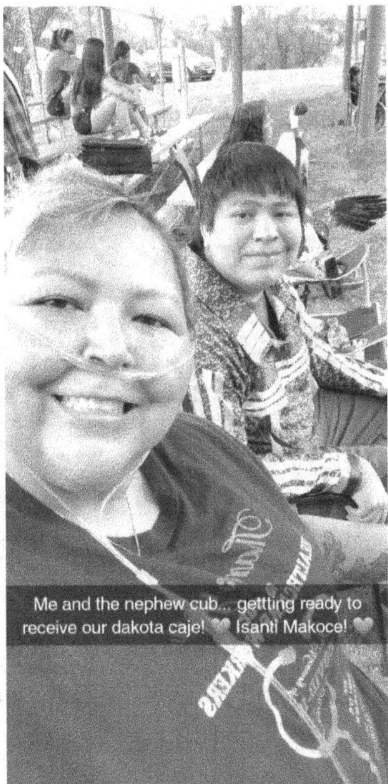

Figure 25: Isanti Pow Wow 2021

I eventually ran into my cousin Baby Trooper sometime and I was so happy to see him. I hadn't seen him in years. I knew he was praying for me and having healing ceremonies for me. The shadows that were circling me in the shadow room while I was in the hospital were the spirits coming to get me. I had one foot in this world and one foot in the other world. He told me, "I'm so happy that you decided to stay in this world!" He hugged me and went on his way. I teared up because I knew exactly what he meant, and I too was happy that I had decided to stay on this side. It was more important to me now than ever to get my *Dakota C'aje*[9]. I was not afraid to sign a DNR, but we believe our relatives recognize us by our *Dakota C'aje* and I had not received one growing up, only the one I was assigned by birth order. I had been sober nearly a year and I wanted to get my nephew and I our names. My dad set it up for us to have a ceremony as a family. He asked our tribal chairman, Roger Trudell, in a good way, to do our naming ceremony. In June 2021, at our annual pow wow, we had our naming ceremony together:

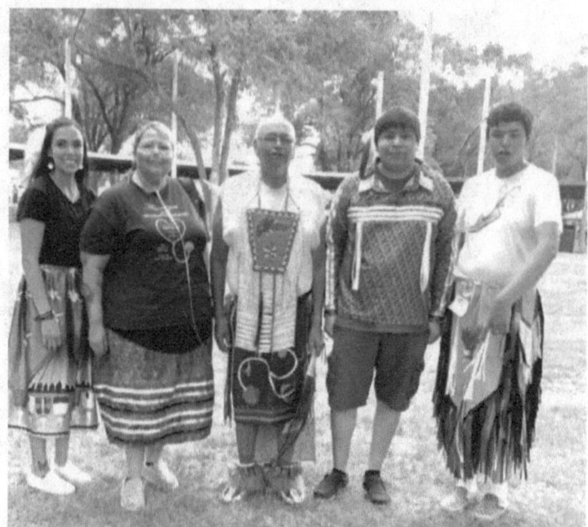

Figure 26: Red Owl Family Isanti Pow Wow
2021 – Naming Ceremony

my dad, myself, my sister, my nephew and my youngest brother. I was thankful to have been honored as a family and receive our *Dakota C'aje* together. I was not strong enough to walk the circle, but I had my mobility scooter and was able to join my family with our honoring around the pow wow arena. Although I was still healing, I felt complete and was now brave enough to walk in either world.

I could tell that I had gained stamina in the Bryan program. I met some great people in the therapy sessions there and one of my favorite people I met was a lady who was in therapy because she had lost her leg. She wasn't in my lung therapy class, but her therapy coincided with mine. She was thin, had long silver hair, and was very pleasant to talk to. She made a point to acknowledge me or say "hi" when she saw me. I learned that she had a twin brother who had passed not too long prior, and it dampened her outlook on her upcoming birthday. I gave her encouragement to celebrate for him and for still being here. I was inspired by her generally pleasant personality and I could tell that she did not see herself as a victim of her circumstances. She showed up every day. She would have her prosthetic leg over her shoulder and came to get ready for therapy. When her prosthetic was on, she walked on the treadmill and was learning to balance her core with the newness of the prosthetic. I never did get her name, but she was such an inspiration to me and my journey to keep on moving. I decided a long time ago to never have a victim-mentality and I could tell she was like me in that manner, which is what drew me to talk to her. She would often give words of encouragement. I also met Vicky, who asked if I knew any "Whipple's" from Santee and I confirmed that was my family. It was such a small world; she was the administrator of the Santee Sioux genealogy page and helped people connect with documents and historical items tracing family roots to Santee Sioux ancestors.

When my twelve-week lung therapy session ended, I asked if I could go through again. The therapists told me that no one usually goes through twice, but I told them that I felt a bit overwhelmed trying to get off of oxygen by myself. I graduated from lung therapy at the end of June or the beginning of July 2021.

I revisited my lung doctor and all my tests showed improvement. He was very knowledgeable about post-COVID therapies and strategies. I told him that I had found out that the University of Nebraska-Medical Center (UNMC) had a post-COVID clinic that had all disciplines needed for post-COVID patients like me: lung doctors, rheumatologists, mental health practitioners, kidney Doctors, and physiatrists. I was on the waiting list to be admitted to the clinic and I shared the email with him and he sent a referral on my behalf. In the meantime, I asked to be sent back through lung therapy and he agreed.

This time, however, LifePointe had a waiting list until September of 2021. I didn't want to wait that long so I asked them if there was another institution that offered lung therapy and they advised me that CHI Health had a lung therapy program. I thanked them and let them know that I would look into CHI Health to see if the wait would be less.

I contacted CHI Health, and they were able to take me in right away. I went in for an assessment and did a six-minute walk test and was able to begin new lung therapy on Tuesdays and Thursdays for thirty-six visits. The CHI lung therapy was more my style and speed. It was an all-around workout and it focused on strength building, whereas the previous lung therapy was cardio-based. Don't get me wrong, I needed the lung therapy at LifePointe to be cardio-based because I was extremely weak. I had to build stamina and strength over twelve weeks to prepare me for the next step in my journey.

Nebraska Medical (UNMC) called and said I was approved for the post-COVID clinic, and I had an appointment set up for July 2021. I was expecting to be seen at UNMC's main campus but when I arrived in Omaha, I was at a primary care doctor's office. Surely, this couldn't be the post-COVID clinic with all of the doctors that I needed to see. The building was small and the same size of my primary care doctor's office in Lincoln, if not smaller. At the registration desk, I told them that I was there for the post-covid clinic, and they looked as though they had no clue what I was talking about, but they had me on their schedule. After a brief wait, I was taken by a nurse to a room where my vitals were taken. I asked about the post-COVID clinic, and she didn't know what I was talking about either.

Finally, the doctor arrived, and I let him know that I felt very confused because I thought I was going to a post-COVID clinic that had studies and all of the disciplines in the same spot for me to be seen by everyone. He advised that he was more or less the "gatekeeper" and that he would refer me to each discipline. I asked what the difference between that and what I got from my primary care doctor in Lincoln was, and I never did get a clear answer. He did refer me to psychology, dermatology, pain management, and speech therapy to help with my anxiety, skin concerns, and COVID brain-oh, and a neurologist. I never did figure out what the post-COVID clinic was, but he was just my primary care doctor in Omaha, and he referred me to things I was concerned with. There was no structure or discipline that led me to believe I was in a COVID study or a long-COVID (aka post-COVID) clinic. The neurologist ordered a CT scan of my brain, and it came back normal. The dermatologist looked over my skin and prescribed ointment for my psoriasis and PsA. The speech therapist worked on my word jumbling, short-term memory loss, cognitive delay and brain fog. The psychiatrist prescribed me some medications to help with general anxiety and post-traumatic stress disorder (PTSD). She recommended that I see a psychologist for counseling, coping and therapy strategies. The waitlist for a counselor was up to three months out at UNMC. I was able to find two counselors in Lincoln and started mental health therapy for my PTSD and anxiety from COVID.

The lung therapy at CHI Health monitored my oxygen and heart rate after every type of exercise. It started with ten sit-to-stands or squats, resistance band exercises to work the arms, and dumbbell weights. I started at eight pounds, which I was very impressed with considering I couldn't lift two pounds in February. Then we would do a weighted carry, one lap around the track, and I think I might have been able to carry ten-pound dumbbells. They would split us up and I was assigned to an elliptical machine for five minutes. It took every ounce of energy I had to complete the full lung therapy session. Then we did stretches and got our last oxygen and heart rate readings. My face was so red from the workout at first, and I sweated profusely. I hated having sweat in my face, so I often wore a bandana that matched my outfit for the day. I used to have to be color coordinated from head to toe-I was a trend-setter.

Lung therapy wiped me out completely. I would have to go home and take a nap or two during the day just to get my energy back. I was still on oxygen full-time at home, but I was able to make dinner without pulling a chair into the kitchen to sit on while I stirred or browned the hamburger. I could see progress in a positive direction.

I was on a great path to regaining some of my functionality, but I did not have a realistic idea of when I would be ready to go back to work full-time or when I would regain my functionality completely. I thought I would be able to go back to work in the fall or October, but my PCP doctor warned me that I should not try to go back too early and either hurt myself or get myself in trouble with my employer if I wasn't able to perform my job duties. I took her advice, decided not to jump the gun and took my time going back to work. Even though I was building strength and stamina, I had no energy to do anything else. My full-time job was to get better and work on my lungs, strength and stamina so I could continue my progress of walking on my own and maybe one day getting off of oxygen.

In August 2021, I learned a hard truth. My friend and realtor, Jenee Pekarek, invited me out to Branched Oak to go boating. I was excited to be out of the house and since it was such a beautiful day, I agreed to go. We had snacks; I brought my own beverages because I did not know what would be available for our day on the lake and I didn't drink sugar or alcohol. We cruised up and down the lake and parked at different spots around the lake. She showed me the parts of the lake that were her favorite and where people camp or party coves. I used to own a boat, so I was happy to be back on the water. We had to use the restroom, and what do you do when you need to use the restroom on a boat? You jump in the lake. She jumped in the lake off to one side and I jumped off the back. I floated away from the boat and relieved myself, then started to wade back toward the boat. It felt so good to be in the water and swimming. I noticed the boat was drifting away, so I started to swim toward the boat. I have always been a great swimmer, but I noticed quickly that this swim took all my energy. It seemed like it took forever to get back to the boat, but it was only about twenty-five feet. I finally reached the boat and took a short break to catch my breath. After a rest, I tried to climb up the ladder and almost got up the first step on the first try, but the ladder was different from the steps I was used to at the pool-it was harder, and a higher climb. I rested and tried again two or three more times before Jenee and her friend finally had to pull me into the boat. I was exhausted and my ego was

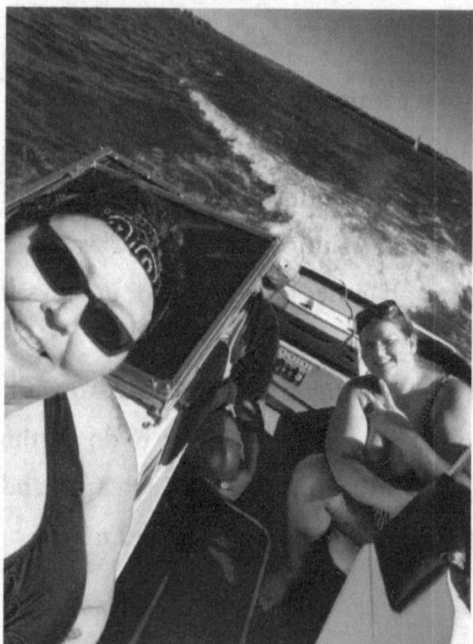

Figure 27: Lake Day Aug 2021

deflated because I thought for sure that I should have been able to make that step. It was a rude awakening that I was weaker than I thought. It was then that

I realized that I was nowhere close to being able to go back to work. It showed me how much work I needed to do before I even considered working. I didn't let on that I was feeling defeated and tried to enjoy the rest of the boat trip. I haven't been on a boat since, but that experience added more fuel to my fire that I needed to regain my functionality and get off oxygen.

From late-September to late-October of 2021, I started to get panic attacks more frequently. I didn't want to leave my house. My anxiety was through the roof. It was coming up on the one-year anniversary since I went into the hospital and never walked back out. It was a stressful time and it seemed like I relived those moments whenever they popped up on my timeline history on Facebook or Snapchat. I started to see my mental health counselors and they told me to not look at the anniversary as a bad time, but to celebrate it because I had survived. That was easier said than done.

I was on long-term disability and was receiving about 60% of my income and was expected to pay for my health insurance out of that portion. The loss of income was definitely felt across the board. My hospital bills piled up, plus all of the handicap equipment that I needed. I was behind on my mortgage and managed to keep up with my car payments, but was unable to keep up with my credit card debt. I ended up filing bankruptcy to try to save my house and my car. I had never filed bankruptcy before, but it was a very long, tedious process with a ton of paperwork. I thought I had my budget and financials organized and prepared nicely in a spreadsheet, but that was nothing compared to all the paperwork that I had to find and provide to my lawyer. I had to pay my lawyer a flat $1,400 retainer which also added to my deficit, but at least I knew there would be a light at the end of the tunnel.

My CHI lung therapy came and went quickly. Therapy wiped me out completely and I would sleep a lot. I knew I had progressed, but it still took a toll on my energy levels.

I told the CHI respiratory therapists that I wanted to go back through lung therapy again and I was met with the same disbelief as the Bryan therapists when I wanted to repeat that program. It wasn't common for people to want to go back to therapy, but I still found it daunting and scary to try to get off of oxygen on my own. I told them that I was going to visit my pulmonologist and see if he would send me back again.

CHAPTER FIFTEEN

ONE YEAR AND COUNTING

I have never been one to have a victim mentality, but the anxiety and PTSD were prominent and new to me. I started mental health therapy in October to prepare for the one-year anniversary of my trauma. One of my therapists recommended that I focus not only on the traumatic event, but to celebrate being alive for another year. I struggled with that, and I still struggle with it today. How can I celebrate when so many did not survive COVID another year? Don't get me wrong, I am more than ecstatic to be alive and I learned to celebrate life every day. I am very happy to be here.

My birthday is October 2nd, and I did not feel like celebrating in 2021. It was close to the one-year mark since I had started my battle with COVID, but I had my nephew at home, and it was not just me anymore.

Pre-COVID, I took my nephew out to HuHot, his favorite place to eat, for his eighteenth birthday. It was within the first year that he lived with me. I made sure to tell him, "No matter what happens in life, and if I teach you nothing else but this, I want you to know that you must learn to celebrate you. Learn to celebrate your accomplishments and be proud of how far you have come and all you have done to get to this moment, right here, in your life. You and I don't have parents that celebrate for us or throw us parties, so we must learn to celebrate on our own because you deserve to be celebrated. I will always try to help you celebrate for as long as I'm here! I love you! Happy Birthday!" I was so proud of him because he had graduated high school that year. If I had taught him nothing else, I wanted him to learn that lesson. It is so hard to be on your own and it can be a very lonely road. I have been through it and still go through it.

It was my forty-third birthday and I had been home from the hospital for a little over ten months. My nephew asked me what kind of birthday cake we were having for my birthday, and I told him that I hadn't thought about it and probably wasn't going to get a cake. He then told me that he was going to make me a cheesecake for my birthday. I considered my anxiety and reluctance and decided to have a nice dinner with family because my nephew wanted to celebrate. It was a small gathering and last minute, but I enjoyed it as much as I could, even as I was fighting through high anxiety. We came home and enjoyed his homemade cheesecake. I was glad that I celebrated my birthday because I wanted to be consistent in the lessons that I was teaching him. I wanted to be for him the person I needed when I was his age. He taught himself how to make cheesecake while I was in the hospital and bought his own pans, and it was the second, best birthday gift I had received because he made it himself.

I forged ahead and continued with my lung therapy and aquatic exercise on my off days. I hardly went anywhere because I was scared of catching COVID again. In my mind, if I caught COVID again, there was absolutely no way that I would survive what I had gone through a second time. I felt like COVID was now a death sentence for me, so I stayed home.

It had been one year since I walked into the ER on October 20, 2020, and never walked back out. My anxiety was high, but my panic attacks subsided to maybe one per week or every other. Never in a million years would I have thought that I would be in a multi-year battle with COVID-19.

November 8th, 2020 was the day I stopped responding, and I almost died on November 9th or 10th. I read memories on Facebook (FB) that I had never seen or read before as they popped up on my one-year memories timeline. Lots of people were offering prayers for support-some were people I knew, or who knew my parents or grandparents, friends of friends and complete strangers. I was moved and humbled with gratitude and appreciation to the point of tears, seeing so much kindness and support in my time of need. I was focused on the anniversary of my trauma, as many people do, and was overwhelmed with anxiety. During that time a friend of mine was in the hospital fighting for her life against COVID-19. She was always on my mind. When she was first diagnosed, she reached out to me because she was scared. We kept in contact in the early days. She knew that I had been down that dark road and wanted words of advice and encouragement. I advised her to stay up and move around as much as possible to try and avoid the pneumonia from settling. During her hospital stay, she told me her mother was admitted to the hospital as well and that she was scared. I checked in on her from time to time, asking how her oxygen stats were. She reported they were in the nineties but one day she said things had a halo and were fuzzy. I told her to keep an eye on her oxygen and vitals. I wanted to tell her to try and avoid the ventilator, but I didn't because I didn't want to overstep a boundary-everybody views things differently. I figured that the medical team had far more knowledge of COVID-19 than me and there should have been improvements in care since it had been an entire year and they now had COVID vaccinations. When I had COVID there were no vaccinations or knowing what we know now. I thought the doctors surely had a better handle on things by now. I have guilt because I didn't tell her what I wanted to-maybe I should have. I went all the way up to ninety liters or more per minute on high-flow oxygen and peaked, but I knew going into my hospital stay that if I went on the ventilator back then, there was a huge chance that I would not come out alive. Then again, I have underlying medical conditions and my odds are always less than the norm. I don't know if my friend had underlying conditions, but while she was on the ventilator, her mother died. Not too long after, my friend lost her battle with COVID-19 while on the ventilator-she was only in her fifties. I wanted the world to be better, and the knowledge and the advancements against COVID-19 to be better.

When I had started mental health counseling for my anxiety and PTSD from my near-death battle with COVID-19, one of the topics I had discussed was how to help my friend when she came out of the hospital, knowing the daunting, lonely battle she would face to regain the ability to walk and go through recovery. I had never anticipated her death, and I took it hard. My therapist told me that everyone is different, and what worked for me is not going to work for everyone. I did all I could by being there and encouraged her when she needed me. I carried that with me for a long time and I continue to carry my friend in my heart.

I'm not sure if I have survivor's guilt, but I wonder why I was fortunate enough to survive. I don't see anyone out here with my circumstances or anyone to compare my progress to. I felt like I was throwing darts in the dark trying to gauge when I would be well enough to go back to work. As hard as I worked, and as far as I had progressed, I was still not in good health-but I continued to do everything in my power to keep moving forward. I often said that I was "winning this turtle race."

My bestie received a trip offer through Caesar's properties with airfare and room included for two people for $35 per person with options to Laughlin or Reno, Nevada. We had visited Laughlin in late August 2020, amidst the COVID pandemic, so we decided to go to Reno, Nevada. We flew out of Omaha on October 20th and returned October 24th. This was one of the first trips that I took after I got home from my battle with COVID-19. The handicap mobility scooter was such a blessing to have been gifted to me. I was able to ride it all the way through the airport to the actual plane and they stored it underneath the plane. There would have been no way that I was able to travel without that scooter. I was not able to walk through the airport or any of the distances I needed to travel and have a fun, adventurous trip. I was able to take my portable oxygen with me on the plane. I did not want to have to take a bulky bag with me to the tiny restroom on the plane, so I went up the aisle without it. I never considered altitude. When I got back to my seat, I checked my oxygen stats, and they were at 72%, so I turned my oxygen machine on and kept it on. I didn't get dizzy or fall or anything, but I did get a slight headache, which is a sign of hypoxia.

Travel for me required mental preparation. I would never be able to travel like I had before COVID. I had to pack my handicap scooter, my portable oxygen, my sleep apnea machine, and my clothing, and travel necessities, including all my medication. There was absolutely no way I could have traveled by myself to navigate through the airport with all my medical equipment and my luggage. I was saddened by the new realization of what the rest of my travel years could possibly look like. Would I ever be able to simply hop on a plane by myself and go again? The uncertainty is what saddened me after being so independent for so many years.

I was still on long-term disability (LTD), which was only paid once per month and supposed to be paid five business days prior to the end of each month. I had to follow up periodically, every three months, with my doctor to assess whether I was ready to go back to work. I received a text that my LTD payment would be released on October 26th, 2021. The date passed with no payment. I finally called the LTD insurance company and found out that they had denied my claim despite my doctor's recommendation that I was not ready for work. The insurance company said, according to my oxygen needs, I should be able to sit upright for eight hours and return to work full-time. I had to file an appeal. They said because I could navigate stairs and get up from a chair, I should have no problem getting back to work. In my appeal, I stated that they were not taking my entire well-being into consideration. I let them know that my improvement in oxygen needs was not the only health issue I was facing due to COVID. I went to my psychiatrist and my mental health therapists and asked for a general letter of what I was being treated for, which was anxiety and PTSD from COVID. I also stated that I had RA, PsA, and PsO. I was in physical therapy, aquatic therapy and speech therapy. My oxygen needs may have been less, but what kind of life would I have if all I could do was work and sleep? I told them that I was working on building stamina and strength to stay awake for a full day. Any activity took more energy now because my lungs were working harder. I was also combating brain fog, word jumbles-where my words were in the wrong order-and cognitive delay. It took them a long time to review my appeal.

Meanwhile, I had zero income for the foreseeable future. I basically had come from nothing, and had gone without food, heat and electricity before. I knew how to survive, and I could live on cereal, milk and bread if I had to-I had done it before. This time was different, though; it was no longer just me. I had my nephew and my pets to consider. I applied for food stamps for the first time in my adult life. I applied for emergency assistance right away and was approved for

Medicaid, food stamps and energy assistance. I was so thankful that they have those programs available for emergency situations like what I found myself in. We were going to be fine, we had food stamps and energy assistance. I received $250 per month for food stamps.

I am so glad that I had started counseling by the time the LTD insurance company decided abruptly to shut off my only source of income. I went with no income from October 2021 to February 2022. It seemed like all I did during that time was fight different battles; it was all overwhelming and I had no control over any of it. I couldn't file for unemployment or Social Security disability because I was still employed full-time. My employee advocate helped immensely during that time and recommended that I apply to the Employee Relief Committee for emergency assistance.

I visited Dr. Reichmuth for a follow-up and all of my breathing scores showed improvement again, he was convinced that I wasn't done healing. I let him know about my disappointing experience with the UNMC's "post-COVID clinic" that did not exist. He not only sent me back through lung therapy again, but referred me to a physiatrist. The physiatrist was very knowledgeable about COVID and post-COVID and I liked her right away. She sent me to physical therapy, aquatic therapy and speech therapy at Madonna Rehabilitation so that I wouldn't have to drive all the way to Omaha. It would take time to get all the therapy set up with my health insurance company and I had to wait a few weeks.

My gym membership at Genesis Health Club, formerly known as Prairie Life Fitness, was put on hold since I was unable to afford it. I no longer had the intense workout of lung therapy to keep me active until insurance approved my third round of lung therapy. My friend, Tommy Arsiaga, had seen one of my posts about being down on my luck and he invited me down to Southside Boxing Gym. I took him up on it and took my nephew with me just in case I passed out or had a panic attack. I had never walked or stood for more than ten-minute intervals. I instructed my nephew, if I fainted, passed out, or had a panic attack, not to call 911, just to turn my oxygen up and make sure I woke up within a minute and did deep breathing exercises. I had my portable oxygen backpack on with my workout headband, a mask, and we used their equipment the first day. We were taught how to wrap our hands. Then we were taught to jab with the left hand in three-minute intervals, with a thirty second break. I made it forty-five minutes that first day without passing out or having a panic attack, but I was spent. I was so proud of myself, though; it was a tough workout that worked on my breathing. My legs and arms were jelly. My nephew and I started to go on Mondays and Wednesdays from 5 PM to 6 PM, before the boxing classes started, because I was just there to work on my lungs and couldn't do more than jab and move. Tommy told us to use some of the other equipment, but

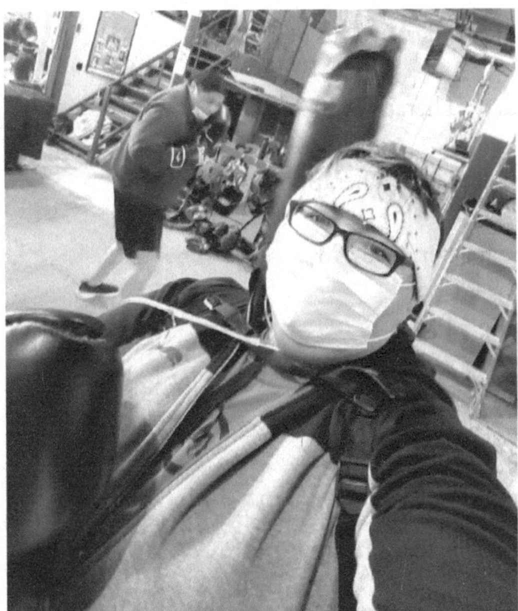

Figure 28: Southside Boxing Gym

we were like fish out of water and didn't know how to properly use the speed bags and stuff. In hindsight, it was very comical once we witnessed the experienced boxers use the equipment that we had tried that first day. It was not the form or method we used, so we just looked at each other and laughed at ourselves. Everyone there was super nice and never asked about my oxygen backpack or my story. I have always been a huge boxing fan and it was nice to watch the young boxers work on growing their talent and track the results of their fights. Coach Tommy and Big E gave us pointers on form and new exercises. I jabbed with my right once in a while and coach Tommy would yell at me, "LEFT ONLY!"

I started lung therapy again at CHI Health for the second time. Lung therapy was on Tuesday and Thursday mornings from 9 AM to 10 AM. I went to Southside Boxing on Mondays and Wednesdays at 5 PM. Then, when I was approved to start physical therapy, aquatic therapy and speech therapy, they were scheduled on Mondays, Wednesdays or Fridays. My schedule would look something like:

- Monday:

  - Physical Therapy 8 AM

  - Physical Therapy Plus 8:30 AM

  - Aquatic Therapy 9:30 AM

  - Mental Health Therapy 12 PM

  - Speech Therapy 2 PM.

  - Boxing 5 PM

- Tuesday:

  - Lung Therapy 9 AM

  - Mental Health Therapy 2 PM

- Wednesday:

  - Boxing 5 PM.

- Thursday:

  - Lung Therapy 9 AM

- Friday:

  - Physical Therapy 8:30 AM

  - Physical Therapy Plus 9AM

○ Aquatic Therapy 10 AM

I napped a lot during those times because of my busy schedule not to mention all the financial stress I was under and the appeal with my LTD insurance company.

My living room floor cracked during the fall. It was the concrete slab underneath the carpet that cracked, and there was about a half inch to an inch drop between one side and the other. I also noticed that my second story wall moved as well. In the corner of the wall, the paint bubbled up and there was a gap between the ceiling and the wall. My foundation and my roof needed to be fixed. This was due to the arctic freeze we had in February 2021. I was able to get my insurance to cover a portion of the roof, but they wouldn't cover any of the foundation.

Shit was hitting the fan left and right, and everything had to be a damn fight. My world wasn't crumbling but the world was heavy as fuck (AF). I only had so much energy to fight so many battles. I was overwhelmed and thankful that I was in counseling. I naturally had the ability to prioritize and compartmentalize problem after problem and tackle them one by one due to my superior survival mentality. However, it just took a toll on me mentally and physically. It was exhausting to have to continually advocate for myself at every turn in the road.

I was so thankful to have an outlet, such as Southside Boxing Gym, to help me work on my lungs. It was also a huge stress reliever to punch something, even if it was just a jab. I think my friend gifted me an Amazon gift card, so we were able to obtain our own gloves and wraps and started to go almost every week. I made the mistake of telling my physical therapist that I was boxing in the evening. I explained it was not really boxing because I cannot box. It was just standing upright and jabbing with my left hand while working on my breathing and moving left or right. The PT told me that I couldn't do boxing on the days that I did therapy, which sucked because I felt like I was really getting the maximum benefit by doing both. I understood that she was worried about me injuring myself. I did get dizzy a time or two at boxing, but I learned to slow myself down. Well, as you can see from my schedule example, it was rare that I did not have therapy. My Fridays were usually free, but the boxing gym was only open Monday through Thursday. When the boxing gym opened on Saturdays, I went a few times, but the consistency was no longer there and I missed Southside.

Everything worked out as it was meant to. I did not get paid in October, November, December or January. I applied for emergency assistance through my employer at the end of 2021 and I only applied for what I felt we needed. The bare necessities-help with electricity, car payment, fuel to get back and forth to therapy, car registration, car insurance, internet, mortgage payment and phone. My employee advocate filed my paperwork, and he and my company went above and beyond for us. It was right before Christmastime, and we were approved for everything I asked for help with. The company included extra money for groceries or household items, or whatever we needed-maybe $200-250-and they also gifted me a $500 gift card to Walmart. At the time, I was in survival mode, and I hadn't even thought about Christmas. My nephew and I made the most of it and bought a Christmas ham and taught ourselves how to make mashed potatoes. His friend came to have dinner and spend Christmas with us, like he had the year prior. He told us that was his tradition, to spend Christmas with us, and we told him he was more than welcome.

Christmas went by quickly, we had originally planned on going to my dad's house but that was before the LTD cut off my income, and we just couldn't afford it. We were still welcome but I am old school and too prideful to go anywhere empty-handed. We stayed home and had movie night. Christmas was my least favorite holiday ever since my grandparents passed away. It was always a lonely time of year for me. I never really felt at home during the holidays like I had with my grandparents. Now that it was just me and my nephew, we had started to make our own traditions, like movie night. I'm glad we made the most of it, and enjoyed teaching ourselves to cook. It ended up being the best Christmas I have had in a very long time.

New Year's Day arrived, and it was cold in the house when I woke up. I thought maybe my nephew had turned the heat down or something. His maternal grandfather is from Alaska, so I tell him he's part Eskimo and tease him about always making it cold for me. When I went downstairs the heat was on, but it was sixty-five degrees in the house. It was the absolute worst time for my furnace to break. Every heating and cooling place I called wanted hundreds of dollars just to show up at our door, and then we were required to pay holiday and overtime wages per hour, which was not cheap. New Year's Day was on Saturday, January 1st, 2022, and I would have normally waited until the holiday was over, but Monday was too far away. My dad went to college for HVAC, so I called him. He told me to check some things on the furnace. I am very adept at hands-on, do-it-yourself, and fixing things, so I understood what he was explaining to me. However, I was only functioning at about 40% of my usual abilities, and if I got on the ground, I wasn't sure if I would be able to get back up. I called my nephew downstairs and let him know our furnace was out and asked if he could come help me look at it. I figured I could teach him a few things with my dad's help. We walked into the laundry and furnace room, and he asked, "Which one is the furnace?" I was surprised that he didn't know but, then again, I was always fixing things with my grandpa or my dad, and I don't think he had had the same opportunities that I had. I told him the water heater is the circle one and the furnace is the rectangle one.

We were able to get the furnace door off and run a test that is programmed into the furnace with the instructions from my dad, and there were some printed instructions on the furnace door. We were looking for the limit switch, but my nephew could not find it and I could not help from where I was standing. We gave up. However, I am not one to *actually* give up. When my nephew went back upstairs to his room, I grabbed my tool bag and got on the floor with some difficulty. I laid down by the furnace and took the door off. I found the limit switch and took it off. I took a picture of it and sent it to my dad. He confirmed that that was the part that I needed, according to the tests we ran earlier. I called everywhere to see if I could find the part, but nobody was open due to the holiday. I called the various heating and cooling companies back to see if they would just sell me the part. All of them said no. Finally, I found a company that was not charging holiday or overtime hours-he wouldn't sell me a part either, but assured me he had some in supply. I confirmed I would hire him and he came to the house within fifteen to twenty minutes. He sounded the most affordable, because I had only a couple hundred dollars-the extra money my company had sent us for groceries and stuff. While he was inspecting the furnace, he was going to try and start it, when I said "I think you will need this," and handed him the limit switch that I had taken out. He reinstalled it, and told me what I already knew, that that part had burned out. He said he had one in the truck, so he left and came back in with a limit switch, which wasn't exactly like the one I had handed him but was similar. He replaced the furnace cover, tried to start it, but took it off again immediately and said the fuse was blown. He lectured me about changing the furnace filter and uninstalling parts and blowing fuses. He put a new fuse in and put the furnace door back on and tried to start it again, but the fuse blew again. So then, he took the new limit switch out again and saw that it was touching metal and that was what was causing the fuse to blow. He modified the part he had installed, to prevent it from touching metal and blowing the fuse again. I wanted to say, "I didn't blow the fuse, *you* blew the fuse." I knew that when I took the furnace door off, as a safety feature, it wouldn't allow the furnace to start, so there was no way that I blew the fuse, but I didn't tell him that I knew that-I was hoping to get a discount. He was only at the house for maybe fifteen to twenty minutes. The time would've been shorter, if he hadn't blown two fuses. He charged me $50 for the install and $120 or $130 for the part. If the parts store was open, that part would have cost me less than $20. I was glad he didn't charge me for the fuses he had blown. The total bill was less than $200 which was all that I had. Even though he charged me a ridiculous amount for the part, I was happy to have heat for my house and my family again.

I hardly left my house due to my anxiety level and the COVID risk was still high in Lincoln. The city of Lincoln published a COVID Risk meter every week. I didn't have much money, but I finally won my appeal with my LTD insurance company. I received my booster shot on January 31st, 2022, my fourth Moderna shot overall. It gave me a little confidence and it was extremely hard to get myself to go out of the house because I thought if I caught COVID-19 again, there would be absolutely no way I was going to survive what I had gone through twice. I stayed home, unless I was going to therapy or meeting a friend for coffee. The mental anguish of thinking I might die if I caught COVID-19 in public again was exhausting and overwhelming.

In February 2021, I went to shoot pool league to get my games in because the deadline to qualify for tournament eligibility was fast approaching. Just my luck, there was a sick person on the other team. I asked him if he had COVID and he said he could not have COVID because he had just had it two weeks prior. He would sniffle and sneeze and wipe his snot and hands on his jeans or shirt and did not wash his hands before touching the chalk or table. I was extremely paranoid, so much so that my anxiety was almost to panic attack level. I used germX every chance I got. I did the 1-5 grounding exercises and deep breathing exercises. I was scared and wanted to leave and go home but I knew I had to finish the league night. I don't think anyone really understood my anxiety-it is hard to explain if you have never had anxiety. I didn't trust anything he said because I had active COVID for over thirty days before. I was up-to-date on my vaccinations and booster shots, and had just had my fourth shot the week prior, but I still thought that if I caught COVID again I would surely die. I had been confined to my house for the longest time and then, the one night I showed up to pool league, there was an ill, symptomatic person there. I fist bumped and did not shake anyone's hands-I did that regardless of if I thought someone was ill or not. My days of shaking peoples' hands were over long before this fateful night.

Over the next few days, I had a scratch at the back of my throat, and I thought "Great! That guy got me sick!" If you wonder, why didn't anyone else get sick? I have no immune system (luck of the draw, I guess) and COVID seems to have it out for me. Pool league was on Tuesday night; by Friday night, I had messaged my dad and told him I got sick from pool league and that my symptoms were a scratchy or itchy throat and congestion. He told me that I had better get checked for COVID-19 because those were the exact symptoms that my stepmom had and she tested positive for COVID-19. *"Great!"* I thought, *"Now I am surely going to die!"* I didn't tell him that, but I made an appointment and went to CVS for a COVID-19 test. I thought CVS had a drive-thru testing site but they told me that I had to go into the building to get tested. This was the same CVS where I had fallen, when I had first come home from the skilled nursing facility. I sat outside in my car debating whether to go in. First, if I did go in and I didn't have COVID, who else was in there and what if they had COVID, I did not want it. I was definitely trying not to die. Secondly, if I did go in there and I did have COVID, who else was in there-I did not want to give them COVID. My anxiety was taking over. Finally, I masked up and decided to go in. I walked through the store to the COVID testing area and there was no wait. I walked in the door and sat in the small room where six-foot-social distancing was nearly impossible. Thankfully, I was the only person there. The clinician administered a rapid COVID test and told me the results would be available in about an hour on the website. I retreated back to my house and my phone buzzed with a notification from CVS: results available. I logged in and the results read, **COVID-19 positive**. My fate was determined; I laid on the couch and wrapped myself in a blanket, like a burrito with only my face exposed with my mask on, waiting to die. My nephew came downstairs and I said, "Lil Beau, can you watch the puppies? I have COVID and I am going upstairs to quarantine." He said with surprise and disbelief, "Really? Yeah, I can take care of the puppies."

I went upstairs and laid in bed, drowning from my thoughts and anxiety, when eventually the thought popped up: *"Well, it doesn't feel like I am dying."* Then a lightbulb went off! Aren't I supposed to get monoclonal antibodies because I am in the high-risk category? I googled Bryan Urgent Care and called to ask them about the antibodies. They advised that I did qualify but I needed a positive COVID test. I told them that I had a positive COVID test from CVS. They would not accept CVS tests, it had to be a test in the Bryan network, and she advised that they were booked for the rest of the night. I asked for the first available appointment in the morning. Thankfully, I had kept apprised of COVID and COVID treatments to know that I was eligible for the monoclonal antibodies. Maybe I was not going to die after all. The next morning, I woke up and went to Bryan Urgent Care for a COVID-19 test; it also came back positive. Then I asked, "How do I get the antibodies?" They advised that they already sent a referral to the Infusion Center and someone would call me to make an appointment for me on Monday. I thanked them and went back to my quarantine. I had been working on letting things be, but it was a learning process for me. I was getting used to letting things work themselves out instead of trying to control the outcome. My nephew took great care of me and brought me meals and water. Monday arrived, and I received a call from the Infusion Center; they were able to get me in right away at 10 AM for the antibody infusion. The infusion itself took thirty minutes and then I was able to go home. I only had to quarantine for five to seven days. My second fight with COVID-19 was mild and I called it "COVID 2." Have you seen the movie *Short Circuit*? "JOHNNY 5 ALIVE!!! NO DISASSEMBLE!!!" I wasn't dead yet, so I wasn't done yet!

It took going through "COVID 2" and all the mental anguish of thinking that I was going to die, the anxiety and PTSD, for me to believe and understand that COVID-19 did not have to be a death sentence for me. The vaccinations and supplemental treatment for high-risk patients like me seemed to actually work. I just needed to be apprised of the treatments, vaccinations, boosters and risks. I had to be knowledgeable about everything COVID, a subject-matter expert. I couldn't believe that there were citizens in America that thought the coronavirus was a hoax, fake news, vaccinations with tracking chips and all kinds of malarkey. I was living proof that the vaccinations and boosters indeed worked and did what they were supposed to. They did not prevent COVID-19 but they prevented me from dying or being hospitalized. The dramatic difference between my first battle with COVID-19 and "COVID 2" was such a relief. The weight of death, or thinking I would die every time I walked out my door, was gone. I encouraged those close to me to get vaccinated because I had witnessed the worst of COVID-19 and as long as people were still dying, there was a need to stay informed and up-to-date on vaccinations and boosters so I could continue life.

Since I knew I was no longer dying, I decided to live. I booked my first concert at Red Rocks Amphitheater, outside of Denver, which was on my bucket list. I was able to buy four front row seats to see Whiskey Myers on June 6th, 2022. They were handicap accessible, so I was able to travel with my scooter. I didn't even know who was going to attend with me, but I was sure I would be able to find someone. The tickets were non-transferrable. I had already booked a trip to Las Vegas for Memorial Day week. I would fly into Vegas on May 29th and would fly into Denver on June 5th for the concert at Red Rocks on my way back to Lincoln.

There was so much I wanted to try and do and see. I wanted to get back to living. I continued to work on my lung therapy and physical therapy so I could go back to work.

CHAPTER SIXTEEN

BACK TO THE LAND OF THE LIVING

I was approved for a loan through the city to help pay for my foundation and my roof repairs, and they were able to tack it on to the end of my mortgage loan so my payments would not increase. My total loan was for $20,000 to fix the foundation. I tried to go back to work part-time at the end of February. I was only able to work up to two hours per day before I was so tired from work and therapy that I would need to take a nap to reenergize. I tried to manage all the therapy, work and family without napping during the day, but it was very difficult in the beginning. I struggled for the first few weeks but eventually my need to nap was less and less.

The roof to my townhouse was repaired in March and I agreed to a bi-annual roof and gutter cleaning contract because I owned a flat-roof and it needed to be cleaned in the spring and fall.

I paid a friend's handyman to rip out our carpet. I hired a foundation company to drill five support piers to fix the foundation. The foundation company put a plastic barrier to block off the living room where the support piers were going to be installed. They put plastic down on the floor and ceiling-it looked like a "Dexter Morgan" room. I had physical therapy that first construction day and left them to work on my house. When I arrived back at the house, I noticed they had parked their big trucks on the main street closest to my house. When I walked in to see their progress, I was talking to them through the plastic, which was thick so it was hard to see through it clearly. They had made significant progress that first day and I could tell there were piles of dirt on the living room floor. The team leader explained that they were in the process of digging down so many feet to install the foundation piers and that things were going great.

I said, "That all sounds great, but how did you guys get all that equipment here?"

He replied, "With our trucks parked on the street."

I replied, "There are no trucks outside, did you happen to leave the keys in them?"

He replied, "Yes, but not by your house, on the main street."

I said, "I just came from therapy and there are no trucks in my parking lot or on the street."

Then the taller guy asked, "Are you serious?"

I said, "Yeah, man, there are absolutely no trucks outside, I think someone stole your trucks!" Then, without another word, the taller guy turned on a dime and bolted like he was going to chase the trucks down.

I had to yell, "WAIT! I'm totally joking!"

Thankfully, he heard me and stopped. We all got a good laugh out of it. In hindsight, I should have let him run all the way around the complex-it might have been funnier. After that lightened the day, I went upstairs to my room. Later in the afternoon, I went out to another therapy appointment and noticed that they had moved one of their trucks further down the street so it would be within their view and they must have grabbed their keys. I just smiled and laughed and thought to myself, *I bet they never leave their keys in their trucks again.*

They drilled on the inside of my house and there were heaping piles of dirt on the floor in my living room. That night I let my puppies out to potty out the front door, which was unusual for them. We have a tie out chain in the back and normally tie them up so they do not run away. The living room was sheathed off, with a giant dirt pile blocking access to the patio. I was not quite sure where I had last put the walking leashes, since our house was under construction. I just let them out without their leashes. They were really good at first and went potty on the shrubbery in our walkway, but then they both took off on a deadass run! The little delinquents ran like they were running from police dogs or something. I didn't have my oxygen on and couldn't run after them. Wrigley eventually came back to the front door. Fenway, my little Sour Patch COVID baby eventually came back, but he was barking at the back patio door. I called him our Sour Patch COVID baby because we had adopted him in March 2020, during the pandemic, so he only knew me and my nephew. That is where COVID baby came from. Then he is defiant and cute, he can be super sweet and cuddly, he even knows how to smile, but he only shows my nephew and me his sweet side. He gets anxiety when he meets new people and he's super protective so he growls at them, and that is why he's a Sour Patch, like the candy commercial. Fenway didn't know what "go to the front door" meant or that the entire living room was wrapped in plastic and we couldn't get to him. He couldn't hear me when I went out the front door and yelled for him. I finally had to ask my nephew to go get him. My nephew put on his shoes and coat and had to walk all the way around our complex to get Fenway. Thankfully, the foundation work only took two days and my puppies were able to go back to their normal routine.

When the foundation was completely repaired, we had four patches of new concrete that had to dry-one patch was larger and covered two piers. They put concrete filler or sealer in the cracks that were caused by the damage. The floor was uneven, and I didn't anticipate how unlevel the floor would be. I thought that the foundation repairs would fix the floor and, when they lifted the foundation, I thought that would also fix the gap in the ceiling on my second story. I was wrong. I didn't want to reinstall the carpet because of the traffic of my pets. I received my backpay from my LTD insurance company and bought laminate floor planks with an easy lock system. I had to buy self-leveling cement so we could level the living room floor.

I decided that we were going to install the floors ourselves instead of hiring someone to come and do it for us. I had always been very handy and knowledgeable about tools and how to fix things. I thought it would be a great learning opportunity for my nephew, and I would teach him how to use tools and install a floor. My Grandpa and my dad were both handy, and I was always fixing or working on something with one of them when I was growing up, and I wanted to pass that on to my nephew. I told him, even if we tried it and failed, better to have at least learned and have tried, than to not have tried at all. I wanted him to know that we could do things and learn things to be independent and to take care of our own house, even if we fail. Failure is okay, as long as we had given it our best and got up and tried again. And if we messed it up really badly, then we could hire someone.

Our front entrance had ceramic tile that was installed with cement grout. I thought it would look weird to have wood planks all the way through the first floor except the entrance, so I decided to tear out the tile. I often forgot that I was not at 100% functionality and may never be at 100% again. I considered myself to be at 50% capacity when we started the floor project. I sat either on the bottom step by the front entrance or my garden wagon and hammered and chiseled as much tile as I could. It took two or more weeks to get the stubborn tile and grout removed. We bought an angle grinder without the vacuum attachment-I do not recommend it. Once the tile was chiseled off, we used the grinder on the grout and smoothed out the surface. Without the vacuum attachment to suck up the dust, the entire house was covered in a cloud of dust. It was so dusty, the dogs stood by the back patio door and wanted to go outside. My nephew and I had masks on, and I tried to blow the dust out the front door with the shop vac but that idea didn't do much good. Once we were finished and the dust had settled, we looked at each other with our dust-colored hair and my nephew coughed slightly. When he coughed, a small cloud of dust formed off of his mask. I could not stop laughing, it looked so funny. We swept and vacuumed but there was dust everywhere.

When we finished removing the front entrance tile, we decided to do a trial run on the self-leveling concrete to hide any blemishes we may have missed with the angle grinder. We did one pour, and it only took twenty-four hours to set up and it looked good. It was a little bit higher than the original floor, but there were so many chips in the concrete, either from age or the previous owners. We shimmed it and put cardboard down, so it leveled down when we installed the flooring.

We took a break after the front entrance concrete was poured. I took my nephew to the Denver March Pow Wow in mid-March 2022. We met my dad and sister there. It was the biggest pow wow he had been to. There were plenty of vendors there and we got some cool merchandise. Most importantly, we went to watch my dad dance. My dad was a men's northern traditional dancer and I loved to watch him dance. We had a good, fun, short trip and my nephew did great driving in Denver. I was glad that I was able to take my handicap scooter with me, otherwise I would not have been able to walk the far distances or even get into the Denver Coliseum.

When we returned from our vacation, we started back on our flooring project. I asked my *h'unka*[10] brother, Kyle, to help us pour the living room. When he arrived, he told us that we didn't have a mixer and the power drills were not meant to mix concrete. We poured what we could but we did not have enough supplies to do the entire floor; we were only able to cover the edges. That first pour had to sit for twenty-four hours before we could pour another layer.

The second pour went better, mainly because I bought an actual mixer. I had to rebuy enough self-leveling cement to cover the entire living room plus extra so we did not run out again. I hired two people I found on FB to help us mix and pour cement, since I was unable to help much and Kyle was busy. We were able to get the living room poured in two hours with the hired help. It was a production line. I had bought multiple mixing buckets so we could pour and reuse. I was on water duty and put the measured water in the bucket. One guy cut the cement bag open and poured it in the bucket and used the mixer to mix it. Then my nephew and Christian, the other helper, poured and troughed the cement. Christian was very knowledgeable and had poured this type of cement before. He gave my nephew and the other guy pointers and taught them a few tricks of the trade. We waited more than twenty-four hours for the living room to dry because it was 18 ft by 14 ft.

Once the cement had dried, we were able to put down the vapor barrier. Words of wisdom: the red tape didn't stick very well for us-in hindsight, we should have just used duct tape. My nephew thought it was odd that I had strategized our floor plan by sorting the planks. I will be honest, I was expecting six to eight different patterns, but there were more like twelve to thirteen different designs. I sorted them to inspect for damaged boards, and I didn't want similar designs next to each other but more of a random pattern. I got that idea when I watched YouTube floor installation videos.

It took a couple of tries to get started because we had to do a lot of cutting and prepping the boards. The boards that touched the wall had to have their tongue or groove cut off, or the mommy or daddy cut off, so they were flush against the wall or the spacer. At the time, I could not for the life of me remember what they called the end parts, so I called them the mommies and the daddies. From that point forward, we referred to the board we needed and which part to cut off as the mommy or the daddy. It was only after our project was completed that I finally remembered they referred to them as the male or female parts. I sat my nephew down and explained to him, mechanically-speaking and when doing industrial-type work, they called them male or female parts and I am the only one that calls them the mommies and the daddies because of my COVID brain. He understood-he was used to my unusual speech from COVID by then and often had to tell me when my words were jumbled or if I had used the incorrect word. I was not able to repeatedly get down to the floor and back up again. Once the vapor barrier was down, I just stayed on the floor. I had to wear knee pads, wrist braces and elbow pads. I maneuvered around the floor by rolling to the left or right. We started the pattern with half of a plank to begin our random pattern. We had to start on the west wall so that the starter board would have a daddy plank exposed, then the mommy board would hold it in place. We placed spacers along the wall for the first row. (We used samples of laminate flooring that were the same width as our flooring and cut them into smaller pieces to use for the spacers.) We separated the flooring project into two main parts- the living room floor and the kitchen floor, including the entryway-and bought transition pieces to blend the floor sections together.

We were so excited when we finished the living room floor installation. It was a lot of hard work, and we learned from it. The kitchen and hallway went a little bit quicker because we had one successful room under our belt and had experience and knowledge that we didn't have before. It was a lot of hard work to finish the kitchen and hallway as one long single room but it was worth it to have that continuous-flow look. I told my nephew that he would be able to tell his children about his crazy aunt that taught him how to install floors. All we had left was the transition pieces and to reinstall the base boards. Easier said than done-we needed a nail gun.

We had unplugged the stair lift for the flooring project and I decided not to plug it back in so that I was forced to walk up and down the stairs on my own. The stair lift has been out of operation since. I decided to leave it there in case I need it later or when my arthritis gets really bad. My rheumatologist told me that the stair lift would increase the value of my house.

I continued therapy from March to May 2022. I worked on strength and was able to build enough stamina to work four to six hours per day without consuming all of my energy. I worked smarter, not harder. I was able to split my shift to get all six hours in, and that gave me a bit of time to rest and recharge. My company was very flexible and worked with my therapy schedule. It felt so good to be part of the working class, at least more than half-time, and back to the land of the living.

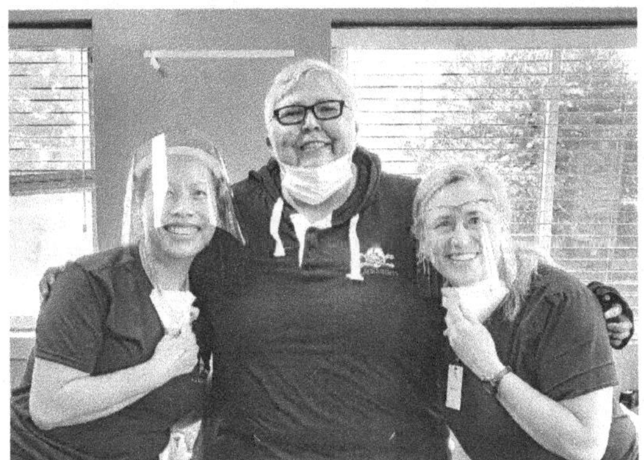

Figure 29: Janet, me and Michelle, 2022

I went back to Ashland to visit my therapists and thank them for helping me get home. It was a coincidence that Janet and Michelle were still there-they had both gone to work at other places and came back to work there at the time I stopped in to visit them. I was so happy to be able to thank them in person and let them know how much their help meant to me. They let me know that I have been one of their greatest success stories.

CHAPTER SEVENTEEN

VEGAS 2022

I became eligible to get my fifth Moderna shot on May 29th, 2022, which was the Sunday that I was scheduled to fly to Las Vegas for the Valley National 8-ball League Association (VNEA) pool tournament. I tried to get the shot one day early, but two CVS clinics in Lincoln didn't know that anyone could get a fifth shot, and then wouldn't give me one because it had to be on the 29th of May, exactly four months after my last shot. The system would not let them enter it on the computer before exactly four months had elapsed. I tried to schedule it online as well and it did not let me make an appointment. Maybe this was my payback from not allowing the nurse to give me blood thinners one hour early. Steadfast in the time frame, I got it and just had to go with it.

Since I could not convince anyone to give me the shot on the 28th, I had to leave earlier for my flight and stop in Omaha to get my Moderna booster. The fifth shot was only available to high-risk people with a compromised immune system. I was alarmed that none of the CVS pharmacy locations that I stopped at were informed that a fifth shot was available to my demographic and the elderly. I was not patient zero. The pandemic had been going on since December 2019. I did not get my first case of COVID until October 2020. There should have been plenty of patients that had received their fifth Moderna shots before me. If they were not informed, I thought the pharmacy should have been the experts to let them know.

My nephew drove me to Omaha so he could drop me off and help me with my luggage. We stopped at a CVS in Omaha, and he waited in the car while I went in to get my fifth Moderna shot. I didn't know this at the time, but some people were calling the vaccination shots "the Fauci Ouchy." I saw a t-shirt that had a large Band-Aid on it and it said, "I got my Fauci Ouchy!" I thought that was pretty dang funny and something I would wear. It didn't take long for me to get my shot. It took longer for me to convince them that I was eligible to get the shot due to my high-risk category. They verified the information on the CDC website before they gave me my shot and signed my vaccination card. I joked and asked if I got a free coffee or prize for filling up my card, like a COVID shot bingo or something. They were not very amused by me, but it can be hard on people when they least expect an informed person like me to test their knowledge.

Once I was finished at CVS, my nephew dropped me off at the airport and unloaded my mobility scooter, luggage, pool cues, and helped me load it all where I could navigate my way to the check-in desk. I had some difficulty and got stuck in the spinning doors with my luggage. Then my luggage was three pounds overweight, so I had to take things out and wear them or carry them. I definitely had to have my oxygen on and with me. It was a lesson learned from my first flight, after "COVID 1" --the altitude dropped my oxygen saturation, which was unexpected.

Southwest Air gave me an extra seat for my portable oxygen, and it was very nice to have it right beside me instead of on the floor or crowded on my lap. I flew to Vegas with no issues. When we landed, I was one of the last people off the plane, so they had time to get my scooter out of the plane storage. I didn't have much difficulty finding my luggage-I always tie colored ribbon on my suitcase so it is easily identifiable, a trick I learned long ago. I am sure I was quite the sight. I was wearing the sweaters and hats that I had removed from my suitcase. I had my oxygen backpack on. I drove my mobility scooter with my pool cues resting in front of me, between my legs, which made it difficult to steer. I drove and steered with one hand, while I pulled and steered my wheeled luggage with the other. It was hard to find a taxi that was handicap accessible, but I was in no hurry and the traffic directors were extremely nice. The traffic lady went almost a quarter of a mile down the roadway to find me a cab. My cab driver was friendly and let me know that if I needed a handicap cab, to call the company and ask for her. I finally arrived at the Flamingo and checked my bags into my hotel at the curb. I navigated my way through the hotel to locate the lobby and registration desk. I checked in and got my room keys, and rested and charged my scooter, oxygen and phone. I unpacked my clothes and was excited to be in Vegas. I was excited to be alive and to have the ability to travel. It was challenging, but I was happy to be able to travel by myself. I had to wait for my bestie to arrive, because she had traveled on a different flight.

It was my first trip to Las Vegas since before the COVID pandemic. I used my flight credits from our canceled trip from 2019, when the world went on lockdown. It was my first trip to Vegas sober. I was excited for my first sober trip; it was going to be different because I would remember the whole trip this time, but also because I was so blessed to have lived and was able to travel again.

I was happy to be there every day, no matter what was going on. During the pool tournament, I had to shoot pool with my oxygen backpack on, but I was still able to shoot straight and won a game or two. I was thankful to be there. I took everything in and everything in stride. This year, we had a five-person team, so we had to rotate someone out or in. I didn't mind, I barely had games to qualify to compete-and I was fine sitting out to cheerlead, as I enjoyed watching my team. I was even more excited when I got to play; even with my backpack I was still a good shot, I just had to own it and take my time. We did very well in the tournament. We made it to the big board and that was by far the best we have ever done at VNEA. I was proud of our team.

Our team dressed up on Wednesday night and went to dinner at Gordon Ramsey's Hell's Kitchen. It was such good food. I had the short ribs and asparagus with a mocktail. That was the first five-star restaurant that I had been to in my life. It was also the first restaurant that I had ever been to that had mocktails on the menu, which I thought was cool and appreciated, since I had stopped drinking.

It was pricey-my bill was about $100 without tip-but most definitely worth the experience, the ambiance and the company.

I am a little scared of heights and had never been on the High Roller, so we went on that while we were there. It was a cool experience to see the night lights on the horizon of Las Vegas. I only got dizzy once or twice, but when I sat down so I would not fall, the dizziness went away. I had made friends in Vegas over the years, and one of my friends, Chris Parker, had recently moved back from Ohio. He was a talented bartender that did all the bottle throws and flips, so we stopped by our favorite bar to see him. They were busy on Saturday night, so we ordered a couple of sodas and a hug, but we forgot to get a picture this year.

Originally, I was scheduled to fly into Denver, my nephew was going to pick me up and we were going to attend the concert at the Red Rocks Amphitheater together, but he was not feeling well. I talked to my friend Vonda, who had driven herself and her grandson to Las Vegas, and asked if I could ride back to Denver with her. I was concerned about her because she had a sinus infection, and I wasn't sure if she was going to be able to make the drive alone. If she said no, then I would just fly to Denver and rent a car. Vonda said I could ride with her and was more than happy to have the company. We were hoping that her antibiotics would kick in and she would feel well enough to attend the concert with me. I canceled my flight earlier that day and our whole team went to the awards banquet that night.

The VNEA 2022 was hosted at Westgate, which was down toward the Sahara but about a block off the strip. On the last night before flying home, we went to the Westgate for the awards banquet. We knew the President of the VNEA board of directors, Marshall Kohtz, and we had a pre-party in his awesome suite. It had a pool table, a bar, and it was one of the nicest rooms that I had seen in Vegas so far. After the pre-party, we went down to the banquet hall. My anxiety was high because of all of the people and the buffet-style dinner, but I thought it would have been rude to skip the banquet and I continued to wear a mask and sanitize my hands. I was worried about my friend with the sinus infections because she could barely keep her eyes open and wasn't feeling well. I think it took all of her energy to attend the banquet. I was hoping she would let me drive the next day.

That night, Saturday, June 4th, we were on our way back to the monorail to the Flamingo hotel. At the entrance of the Westgate, in passing, I saw the owner of the Raiders arrive. I was just cruising in my mobility scooter with my bestie walking beside me and I was like "Hey! Aren't you the owner of the...um." My COVID brain drew a huge blank! He must have thought I was a basketball fan because he answered for me, "the Aces," who were the professional Women's National Basketball Association (WNBA) team that he also owned. I told my friend that my brain had drawn a blank when I had talked to him, but his name was Mark Davis and he owned the Raiders and I loved his cool hair-if he didn't have a unique, distinguishable haircut, I would not have recognized him. He probably gets that all the time, but not many like me, who forget their words mid-sentence while they are cruising by in a handicap scooter. But then again, we were in Vegas.

CHAPTER EIGHTEEN

RED ROCKS OR BUST

Sunday morning, June 5th, 2022, Vonda picked me up and we packed my stuff in her vehicle, and then we went to pick up her grandson. Thankfully, she let me drive-she might have thought I was batshit crazy, but I told her before we left Las Vegas, "I think I was meant to drive you home." I was so excited to drive to Denver because I had never driven to or from Vegas and had never been to Utah. I was enthralled with the scenery and tried to take pics as we went. Vonda slept most of the way. We arrived outside of Denver after dark. We stayed at Blackhawk because it was part of the Caesars properties, and I got free rooms with them. I planned to stay there for the concert as well.

That night, I had a slight pressure headache before I went to bed and thought, if I wake up with this headache, I might have COVID again. That was a sure-fire sign of COVID, the tension headaches. The next morning, I had the same slight pressure headache, but it went away after I took my morning meds, which included a daily pain pill for my arthritis. Vonda still was not feeling well and the plan was that she and her grandson were going to leave me there and I was going to rent a car. I got up to get ready for the day and considered whether I had COVID. Then, we received messages from our three teammates who had flown home the day prior: they all had tested positive for COVID-19. Dang it. I knew for sure at that moment that I had COVID-19 as well, for the third time. I looked up the

Red Rocks Amphitheater policy and it stated, if you were sick, to stay home. I called them immediately to tell them I would not be able to attend the concert that night due to COVID and asked for a refund. They told me that they would put in a request for a refund and I would hear back in twenty-four to forty-eight hours.

Red Rocks was a bust. I checked out early and we packed up the car. I could have stayed and gone to the concert and made it a super-spreader event, but I wasn't that kind of person. If I was able to prevent or protect people from getting COVID-19, I would do that. I decided to continue to drive home with Vonda, and I am happy that I did because I wasn't sure if she would have made the 7.5-hour drive home on her own. We left right away to get home as soon as we could. Vonda felt bad that I was going to miss my concert, but I told her it was only a concert, that there would be other concerts, and that I was hoping for a refund. I was convinced that I was meant to drive her home and repeated it to her. As our trip went on, I became increasingly worried about Vonda's deteriorating health. The headaches she described reminded me of the pressure headaches that I had had when I first got COVID-they were blinding. I let her rest until I almost dozed off while driving down the interstate, then I had to wake her up and switch drivers. I think I took about an hour nap while she drove and when I woke up, I was ready to drive again.

When we arrived back in Lincoln, after seven-plus hours, we dropped her grandson off and then we went straight to her house. I called my nephew to meet me at Vonda's house because she needed to go to the hospital. When we arrived at her house, I hopped out of the driver's seat with the car still running and my nephew and her husband grabbed my luggage and put it in my car. Her husband jumped in the driver's seat and drove her to the hospital.

I went to get a COVID test in the Bryan system and asked for the antibodies again. I tested positive for COVID-19-this was "COVID 3." This time, they prescribed me the antibodies in pill form, aka Paxlovid. The pills tasted terrible and I had to take them for five days. "COVID 3" was mild. I had slight pressure headaches and sticky congestion in my sinus cavity-it was glue-like and felt strange, like I could never get my sinuses cleared. I quarantined for seven days this time and survived "COVID 3."

After quarantine, I realized that I hadn't heard from Vonda, so I messaged her and learned she was in the hospital with clots in her lungs. I went to visit her in the hospital, and I was so happy to see her sitting up. She looked ten times better than when I had last seen her when we got back from Vegas and I was truly worried about her. I told her that I was so happy that we got home when we did and that I knew that I was meant to drive her home. I told her how lucky she was to have caught the lung clots because that was the main risk with COVID-19 and why they had me on blood thinners. If one got loose and went to the heart or brain it could have been fatal. She was so happy that I had driven her home and thanked me. She wanted me to meet her mom, but I had a therapy appointment and was not able to stay long. I told her that I would meet her mom another day and I left.

I never did hear back from AXS, the company regarding my refund request for the Red Rocks Amphitheater. In fact, they never even delivered my tickets. They were supposed to be delivered electronically but when I went to my AXS app, nothing showed up in my history or tickets. I ended up calling them two more times after I got back from Las Vegas, and they told me it was up to the promoter and told me to reach out to Whiskey Myers directly on social media, which I did, but never received a response from them either. At that time, I had limited income and had fought my way through COVID for over a year to see a concert at Red Rocks and to check one item off the bucket list. Then I got hit with "COVID 3" and I couldn't even get a refund, even though I had abided by their policy. It was not like I had a full income or could afford to throw $250 away. I was frustrated and disappointed with the whole process and lack of response. I filed a complaint with PayPal, who was the payment merchant, and I am still waiting to hear back. I am super sad that Red Rocks was putting me through all of this because it was one of my bucket list venues, and I was extremely disappointed in them. There are other musical acts that I would not mind seeing there, but with the poor experience I had with Red Rocks, I do not know if I will ever try to go back or just take them off of my bucket list. How they treated me just didn't sit well with me-the hoops to jump through, and the calls and unnecessary stress to try to get a refund due to COVID, when I followed their written policies.

CHAPTER NINETEEN

THE SHIFT

I wasn't prepared for the profound impact that writing a book would have on me. I gathered all of the medical summaries and notes from my hospital stay and began to read through them. A lot of the information was in doctor speech and I had to look a lot of the terms up. It was as though I was experiencing the five to seven days of critical care for the very first time, since I had no recollection of those days. After I read through all of the notes, I was overwhelmed by what had happened to me. I put the notes and summaries down and had to sit with it for a long time to process the information. I put writing the book off for about six months trying to figure out how I had survived. The very first meeting with my mental health counselor, I told her my story of battling COVID and why I was there and she had tears in her eyes. I hadn't expected that and wasn't sure if that was normal-I had never been to mental health counseling. My friends assured me that meant that she deeply connected to my story.

I talked to my dad and told him the things that I had found out in the notes and told him that I was going to write a book. I didn't know writing a book would be such a tedious process. I was surprised by the time commitment and reliving some of the trauma from my battle with COVID. I finally pieced together the puzzle and it was eye-opening to find how close to death I actually was. I told my dad of my experience when my mother's BP plummeted to the point of life-saving measures and that it was déjà vu as I read the medical notes and realized that I went through a similar experience.

I had a difficult time deciding where in my story to begin my book. I started with chapters that were fresh in my mind and that I knew would be later in the book. I didn't want my book to be about my past trauma and early life. I wanted my book to be solely about my COVID experience. The more I had written, the more I understood that people had to know some of my backstory to understand the decisions that I made. I provided a glimpse of my early life and traumatic experiences just for informational purposes and how that shaped my decision-making. I packed a lot of information in the first few chapters, which could be its own separate book.

In the past eighteen to twenty-four months, I have been fighting COVID and post-COVID. I have also been balancing living with severe RA, learning to live with PSA and PsO, and going through multiple therapies to help me navigate life after COVID.

My fundamental core has changed. I went through so much in such a short period of time-I would never be the person I was before COVID. I used to be inpatient, unforgiving, OCD, body-conscious, unapologetic in the way I viewed the world, it was my-way-or-the-highway. I was quick to judge on instinct and rarely gave people second chances. I had always had zero tolerance for domestic violence, still do-but I handle intolerance differently. My entire outlook of the world is different. I am different.

Being in survival mentality for a prolonged period and constantly thinking I was going to die from COVID, changed me. Having to choose between the lesser of two highly probable death sentences changed my psyche. Going from being prideful on my independent nature-to being helpless and 100% dependent on others has taught me humility. I am no longer ashamed or body-conscious. My biggest fear pre-COVID was being immobile and losing my ability to walk. Facing that fear and moving mountains to regain that ability, strengthened me.

I no longer need to know the outcome, or be in control of the outcome-I let the outcome be as it was meant to be, without my intervention, stress or worry. I have embraced patience as a virtue and I am no longer inpatient. I am more forgiving of others and of myself. I no longer look at the world through tunneled vision, I see beyond the world. I enjoy meeting new people with my new perspective, I feel everyone on this rock has a purpose, even if they haven't yet found it. It's no longer just my way, I can see things from all avenues, learn different perspectives and alternative methods to achieving the same goal.

I am still an optimist. Now, I don't let the little things bother me or irritate me. I don't focus on the negative and don't voice unnecessary complaints. I am happy to be here every single day and make a point to show gratitude at every opportunity. Being around "negative-Nancys" drains my energy because I have to work harder to try to get them to see the positive, or to be fortunate to be alive for another day and in the present. I don't find value in wasting energy on things that are out of my control.

I still trust my instincts first and foremost but it isn't up to me to judge others and never has been. I keep my circle small and simple. When I first quit drinking, it started out as being a sober-friend for someone in need. As time went on, my sobriety became my journey. Unfortunately, drinking is all I knew and grew up with. I started drinking at thirteen to fourteen years of age, which isn't uncommon. I quit drinking, "cold-turkey" on August 26th, 2020. I have been sober for over two years-the longest I have been sober since I was a teenager. It seemed crazy to me that it is more uncommon to be sober than it is to be drinking alcohol. It should've been the other way around. Alcohol is an illusion and it is everywhere. There is so much societal pressure, people ask, "Why aren't you drinking?" Like I need a reason to be sober-I don't. I chose to provide a drug and alcohol-free home for my *tiwah'e*. I enjoy being clear-minded and I don't miss the hangovers or blackouts or making an ass of myself. I like having self-control over my mind, body and soul and providing a safe place for me and my nephew. It doesn't bother me or tempt me to go to bars or establishments that offer alcohol, I just drink water or soda. My sobriety is of great value to me. I'm learning a new way of life and breaking the cycle of alcoholism.

The most notable change that I found is that my world no longer crumbles. The sky no longer falls. I feel like I am on a whole new level of faith, optimism and humility. Even when I was fighting all the post-COVID battles, not getting paid for four months and everything was a fight. My world didn't crumble it, I had internal faith and understanding that everything would work out as it should, in a good way- *"Tanyan aye kte[11]."*

I pride myself on being intelligent and a quick learner but COVID brain fog and cognitive delays made me doubt myself. My speech would often be jumbled, incoherent or completely blank. I had to learn how to slow myself down and to think before I spoke. Writing this book, was difficult because I often couldn't think of the words that I wanted to use or second guessed myself and my vocabulary. It was ever present when I had my book proofread. In retrospect, I should have kept track of how many times the proofreader had to put my words in the proper order, indicate improper vocabulary, or overuse of the same word. It had been an eye-opening experience that I needed to take my time and I have a lot more work to do on my COVID-brain aftermath. My speech has improved but I need to work on slowing my mind down so my pen can keep up.

I am more present, observant and listen more. I take time before I speak and do things with purpose. I still have the same sense of humor. I'm not sure how or why I survived but, I am grateful every day that I am on *kuns'i maka*. I am learning to be okay with not being 100% but strive to regain as much functionality as I can. If you know me, my 50% functionality would put most healthy twenty-year-old people to the test. I am learning to live with oxygen dependency. I am learning to be smarter about my energy consumption and conservation. It takes a lot more work to do simple daily tasks because my lungs now have to work harder to keep up.

I have bad days also. Living with severe RA, PsA and a side of PsO, on top of the post-COVID aftermath, is exhausting. I have days where I am in arthritic pain, battle intense fatigue and mental health days. I am still a hypochondriac and germaphobe, I have to be to survive. I am learning to live with anxiety, PTSD and panic attacks and how to cope with them. I see a mental health counselor and a psychiatrist once per month. There are days when I don't want to leave my house because people are still dying from COVID. Even though, I keep informed on COVID, I don't want to risk having to experience what I went through with my first fight with COVID. I doubt that I could survive that twice. I wear masks in public and people look at me or say things about my mask but my well-being is more important than their opinion or defiance.

I lived in mental anguish from October 2020 to February 2022, thinking that COVID was a death sentence for me. It took catching COVID a second time to show me that with the vaccinations, boosters and antibodies, it no longer had to be a death sentence. I am more willing to leave my house and travel but pick my battles wisely. I decided to live, not just breathe. There is more of the world that I haven't seen but plan to. I have to be responsible and informed and up to date on the latest COVID variant and how to identify and combat it for someone with little to no immunity.

My multi-year battle with COVID and post-COVID shook me to my core and changed my fundamental being. We have a saying in *Dakodiapi*, "*Bdeh'imic'iye*[12]," which means strength comes from within from experience, we have the power to strengthen ourselves from within. I survived the worst COVID had to give. I was injured, almost died, and went through mental anguish, but I am alive and stronger.

COVID is an invisible disease, like many autoimmune illnesses that I struggle with-including mental health. Be kind always-you never know what someone is going through. If you can't be kind-walk away. Nothing is worth giving up inner peace and the power over your emotions. Let it be. *Tanyan aye kte.*

CHAPTER TWENTY

I RISE

COVID-19 took more from me than I can describe in words. The world will never be the same. COVID shook me to my core. I may have died and been revived on November 9th, 2021-I will never know. What I do know is that, eventually, I began to rise out of the flame and ash, like the phoenix, and my soul was set on fire. I have done the unimaginable-I not only survived, but I learned to walk again, breathe again, live again and stand on my own again.

I have fought for my independence my entire life, and I will be damned if COVID-19 was going to take that from me forever. I decided long ago that I would never become a victim and I was not going to start now.

My entire outlook on life has changed. I am lucky to be here and happy to be here every single day. I rejoice in all the love and support that was gifted to me during my time of need and continues to this day.

Humility and patience are virtues that I gained and continue to work on to this day. I am more at peace within my soul, and I am trying to learn to be patient with myself and my healing process. I am winning this turtle race with COVID.

No one knows the far-reaching impact of COVID-19 and the amount of time it takes a person to recover from COVID or long-COVID. If they tell you they do, I call bullshit. So far, I have been in this fight more than two years as of October

5th, 2022. One thing I do know for sure is that I am not dead yet, so I am not done yet!

I encourage you to live life every single day because, oh my, how much life can change in an instant, a day, a week, a month, a year. For better or worse, life is worth the journey. If my story tells you nothing else, I hope it shows you that you can survive the impossible. You must save yourself, advocate for yourself, love yourself, and trust yourself and your instincts. Strive to be the person whom you needed when you were in that moment, on that deathbed, or in despair or praise.

I was in COVID isolation for nearly thirty days or so with no family or friends. I battled a virus that was unfamiliar to everyone and was waging war on me, and the world. Countless people lost their lives to the point that they had to use refrigerated trucks as morgues. For most people, it was a coin toss, as to whether you woke up from being on a ventilator or lost the fight. For others like me, the odds were far less favorable-the odds were in the house's favor.

I was given the ultimatum of intubation or DNR for days on end.

In my situation, they were both death sentences, and I chose Do Not Resuscitate (DNR). Have you ever been given the option of DNR? The psyche that I was in at that time is inexplicable. I am not sure that I can describe it. I hated having to choose between two very probable death sentences and had to mentally prepare myself. I planned my own funeral and wrote it down in a notebook to save my dad and nephew from having to do it for me. DNR might signify giving up-however, in my case, I was simply trying not to die and, in my circumstances, it had the better odds for me.

I never planned on dying, but the options I was given were grim. I wanted an episcopal burial with a combination of traditional drum group and Dakota hymns. I chose "Sweet By and By" in *Dakodiapi* to be my opening and closing hymn. In our culture, we stay with our relatives until they journey to the other side. I had planned a one-night prayer service in Lincoln for my friends who would not make the journey to Santee with me. My wake, funeral, and burial would be in my hometown of Santee. I selected my godchildren and besties as my honorary pallbearers and my bros as my pallbearers. Not my actual siblings, because they would need time to mourn. In our culture, our cousins are our brothers and sisters; and those are the brothers I would have wanted to help me with my journey, in addition to the *h'unka* brothers I have gained over the years. Thankfully, I survived, and my dad and nephew never had to rely on my notebook funeral.

I felt like my oxygen needs had peaked and I was not getting dizzy or fainting. I felt fine other than the fact that my cough muscles hurt. I think it is nothing short of a miracle that I am still here. Even though I chose DNR, I put off signing the DNR by telling them that I didn't think we were there yet, and we would cross that bridge when we got there. No one had anticipated another curve ball thrown at me with an internal hemorrhage. Had I signed the DNR, I would have died on November 9th, 2020, when they had to do life-saving measures to keep my blood pressure up. My blood pressure was 60/42 and plummeted to the point that I went into hypovolemic shock and my kidneys shut down. They had to do life-saving measures and call my family. What saved my life was my will to live and being realistic as to what my risks were and trusting my instincts. When my dad arrived, he also made life-saving decisions to save my life and keep me off the ventilator.

I know that if I had not had a clear mind, I may not have survived at all. I had started my sobriety journey before I had gotten COVID. I needed a clear mind and am thankful for my sobriety every day. I have been sober for over two years, which is the longest that I have been completely drug-and-alcohol free since I was thirteen or fourteen years old. I am not ashamed of my story and unfortunately, my story is not unique. I am surprised that I am still here. I did not have a good outlook on life then and never thought I would live this long. I have been through the thick of it, faced trauma, adversity, culture shock, etc. That does not include my battle with COVID. I needed to break the cycle of alcoholism and lead by example. I was a parent now, and I needed to think about my *tiwah'e* first and show my nephew a different way.

I don't even know where to begin to summarize the survivalist mentality that I had to have to make it out alive. And I am not just talking about COVID.

My story is not a sad story; it is a true story of survivability and unbound determination.

My biggest fear has always been being immobilized and losing my ability to walk. I had always thought that it would be my RA that would leave me 100% disabled and dependent on others. I never anticipated it would be COVID-19.

Once I lost my ability to walk, I was even more fearful that I may never walk again. The severity of my RA is off the charts. I get my nerve ends in my spine burned off with a laser every year because the arthritis in my spine is so painful and hinders my ability to walk. Without the nerves, I have less pain and I can walk. I don't have full functionality in my knees or ankles and feet. Plus, at the time, I was overweight and weighed over 300 lbs. I thought I might never walk again, but I was going to do everything in my power to try to regain my independence and learn to walk and stand again, even if I had failed.

In twenty-eight days at the nursing home, with the help of my physical and occupational therapists, I regained the ability to stand up on my own. I relearned to walk with a walker. They might have thought I was out of my mind, at first, but it just proves that you can do anything if you put your mind to it. I did the impossible and went home by Christmas Eve, 2020.

When I got home, I was not able to lift a 2 lb dumbbell-I had to use a can of soup. I could not walk further than twenty-five feet without stopping for a break or my legs going numb from being so weak. I could not walk up a flight of stairs.

I finished speech therapy. I still use the wrong words sometimes, or jumble them up or draw blanks. The word that I could not think of to describe my headboard was "particle board," like the tabletops at school. I naturally do word-finding and association that can help get me to my point. I have learned to slow down, because my mind moves too fast and that causes a lot of my word jumbles. I have also learned to know when I hit my limit because that is when the cognitive delay and incorrect words or blanks come, when I am exhausted.

Through physical, aquatic and lung therapies, I have not used a walker since March 2021. I can stand up on my own. My mouse muscles can curl 20 lbs. I can bench 55 lb and do 45 lb chest presses. I can leg press 190 lbs. I can walk up and down the stairs. I can walk for more than six minutes. I unplugged my stair lift in March 2022. I have small wins every week or every day. My brother and I went to the casino, and for the first time I went the entire weekend without using my oxygen. Recently, my nephew and I went to the store and I walked to the store without oxygen and without riding the handicap cart. I had to stop for rest and breathing exercises, but I made it. The first time I went down the steps, step-over-step and not one-by-one, I was ecstatic. I can do leg kicks with 5 lb dumbbells in the pool. I went back to work full-time in June 2022. I have built enough stamina that I no longer take day naps. I can go twelve rounds of jabs against COVID-19 at Southside Boxing Gym.

I will likely live with PTSD and general anxiety from COVID-19 for the rest of my life. I have learned to use the grounding exercises in therapy. I still see a mental health counselor monthly. It turns out that I naturally compartmentalize my issues, prioritize them and attack them one issue at a time. Must be one of my survival instincts that has carried me around *kuns'i maka*, for over forty-four winters. I don't think my oxygen hunger will ever go away, but I have learned to get through my panic attacks and anxiety with grounding and breathing exercises and not try to fight them, which makes them worse.

Post-COVID, I am at peace in my soul. I no longer focus on the little things. I try not to let negativity cloud my mind. I am happy to be here every single day. I have learned to slow down and be present.

When I was in my twenties and thirties, I remember my car would break down and my world would crumble because I was too poor to fix it and could not get to work, and I was too prideful to ask for help. Or my lights would get shut off and I would sit in the dark until I could afford to turn them back on.

In June 2022, I accidentally left my keys in my car and forgot about them overnight. It was so hot and humid; my nephew and I did not go anywhere for a day or two until he went out to grab us some ice cream or something. When he came back, he asked,

"Auntie, where is your car?"

I told him it was in the driveway.

He said, "No, it's not there."

I thought he was joking. I told him "Well, if it is not there, someone probably stole it."

My nephew cannot contain laughter so I thought for sure he would break if I asked him for the police department's phone number. So, I asked him to google the Lincoln Police Department's non-emergency number. He looked it up for me and then I figured he would stop me from dialing if he was pranking me, so I dialed it and in a half-panicked voice, he asked:

"Auntie, shouldn't you be calling 911?!?"

I replied "Well, we don't know when it was stolen; it's not like they can go chase someone down the street."

I reported it stolen to the non-emergency number and went outside to double check and to wait for the officer to arrive. I laughed, like "what next?" with hands up in disbelief.

We found the car a day later, less than a mile from my house. It dawned on me that my reaction might not have been typical. I sat my nephew down and explained that when someone's car gets stolen, it can be a very traumatic experience and devastating. I am in a different place in my life, and I am fully insured. I work from home so I don't have an urgent need for a car to get back and forth to work. However, should you ever be around another person that gets their car stolen, do not be alarmed or surprised if they get upset or cry. My reaction was not the norm. He understood.

I use that example because I have found that with all that I have been through in my multi-year fight with COVID, my world no longer crumbles. The sky does not fall. It may crack, but that is when the brightest lights shine through. Those are my people, offering love and support to help build that fire that burns within my soul.

The severity of my arthritis is alarming and I feel that my immune system has upped its fight game and ran amok allowing additional autoimmune illnesses to infiltrate my body for the past two years, which include:

Erythema Nodosum – causes red tender bumps on the shin. Can be indication of other immune disfunction such Sarcoidosis, strep, or cancer. May be a bad reaction to antibiotics. Causes joint pain. Symptoms can be treated.

Psoriasis (PsO) – autoimmune disease, skin regenerates too quickly causing red flaky patches – no cure.

Psoriatic Arthritis (PsA) – autoimmune disease - different from PsO, causes same red flaky skin patches but includes severe joint pain, fatigue – no cure

(Suspected) Cutaneous Sarcoidosis – immune system responding to unknown substance, no cure. Skin lesions, common on scars or tattoos. Can impact the heart, lungs, eyes and other organs.

My arthritis in my spine requires me to have my nerve ends burned off with a laser (radiofrequency ablation) in my lower spine every year just to walk without debilitating pain. My arthritis may start attacking my organs and lungs or become resistant to the medications that I take.

Every day, I continue to fight to improve my lungs and win the turtle race against COVID. I shall never allow my chronic illness or COVID aftermath to define who I am. Currently, I am still oxygen dependent at two liters with exertion, but I no longer need oxygen at rest or when walking at a slower pace. I do all that I can to maintain my mobility and independence.

I may never get off oxygen. I may still need a lung transplant someday. I can be okay with that, but I have decided not to be. I decided that I'm not dead yet, so I'm not done yet. No matter what life throws my way and how many times I get knocked down-I shall continue to rise!

THE AUTHOR

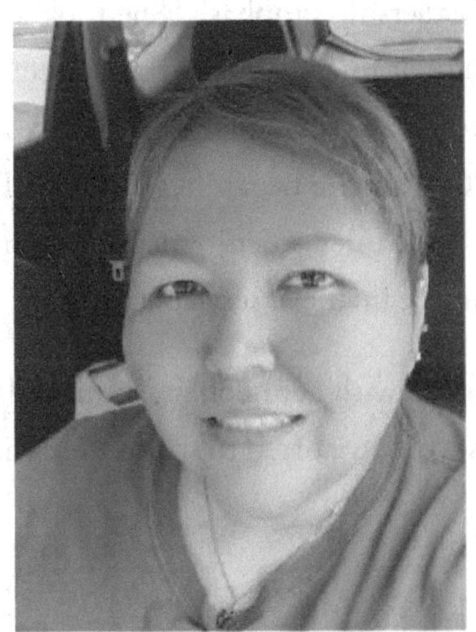

Danielle Red Owl, Tawacin Was'ake Win, is a member of the Santee Sioux Nation and grew up on the Santee Indian reservation in northeastern Nebraska. Danielle graduated from the Nebraska Indian Community College (NICC) in 2000 and transplanted to Lincoln, Nebraska.

She worked at Lincoln Benefit Life Company, later bought by Allstate Insurance, from 2001 to 2007 and promoted cross-functional teams and process improvement.

Danielle attended Wayne State College and received her Bachelor of Science in Business Management in 2009. Danielle worked at Nelnet Inc. from 2009 to 2015, where she made innovative process improvements through system automation. Danielle raised over $25,000 for the American Cancer Society from 2013 to 2017 by hosting annual dart tournaments. Danielle co-founded the Pink Ladies of Lincoln in 2015 with Marshall Kohtz. The Pink Ladies of Lincoln is a non-profit organization that gifts $1000 to people in need battling life-threatening illness, in and around the Lincoln community.

Danielle graduated from Doane University in 2017 with a Master's in Arts in Management with Leadership emphasis. She took a brief contract with her tribe to help modernize their financial reporting system for their revenue-based businesses. Danielle worked as a free-lance Business Analyst with state and federal entities. In 2020, Danielle began her career at PayPal, Inc. as a Senior Business Analyst. She continues to enjoy learning and innovating through process improvements in the financial services industry.

Danielle still lives in Lincoln with her nephew, Beau, and fur babies, Wrigley and Fenway. Danielle travels to Santee often to spend time with family and friends.

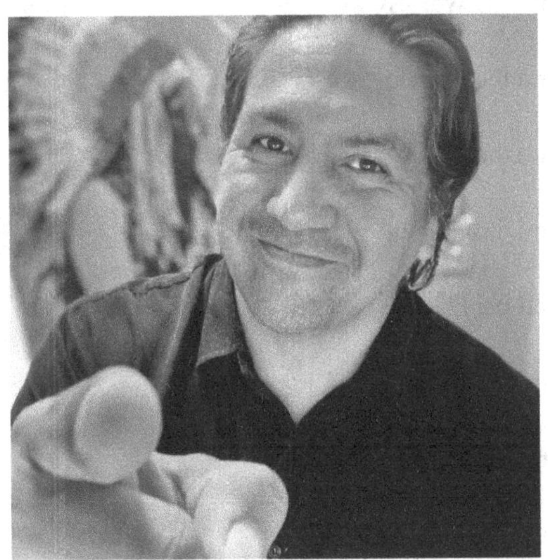

O'MAHK'SIIK'IIMI (aka Jason EagleSpeaker)

Only a few short years after the *Occupation of Alcatraz, the Wounded Knee Incident* and the *Shootout at Pine Ridge Reservation*, a boy was conceived.

Born in Seattle, raised on four reservations and in two cities, Jason EagleSpeaker is both Blackfoot (mom) and Duwamish (dad). He is an award winning internationally published Author, Illustrator and Publisher of over 400 books (with Authors from over 300 First Nations). His hard hitting true stories focus on revealing Indigenous peoples' modern experiences.

You can easily connect with Jason online through social media (Facebook, LinkedIn) or via his website - eaglespeaker.com

NAPI CHILDREN'S BOOKS:

- Napi and the Rock

- Napi and the Bullberries

- Napi and the Wolves

- Napi and the Buffalo

- Napi and the Chickadees

- Napi and the Coyote

- Napi and the Elk

- Napi and the Gophers

- Napi and the Mice

- Napi: The Anthology

GRAPHIC NOVELS:

- UNeducation: A Residential School Graphic Novel

- Napi the Trixster: A Blackfoot Graphic Novel

- UNeducation, Vol 2: The Side of Society You Don't See On TV

LEARN SOME BLACKFOOT:

- My First Blackfoot Word Book

- My First Blackfoot Word Coloring Book

COLLABORATIONS:

- Young Water Protectors

- Sober Indianz

- Indigenous Peoples for BlackLivesMatter

- I Am The Opioid Crisis

- The Great Cheyenne

- The Empowerment of Eahwahewi

- How The Earth Was Created

- My Ribbon Skirts

- Crow Brings Daylight

- Aahksoyo'p Nootski Cookbook

- Indigenous, I Am

... and many many more at eaglespeaker.com

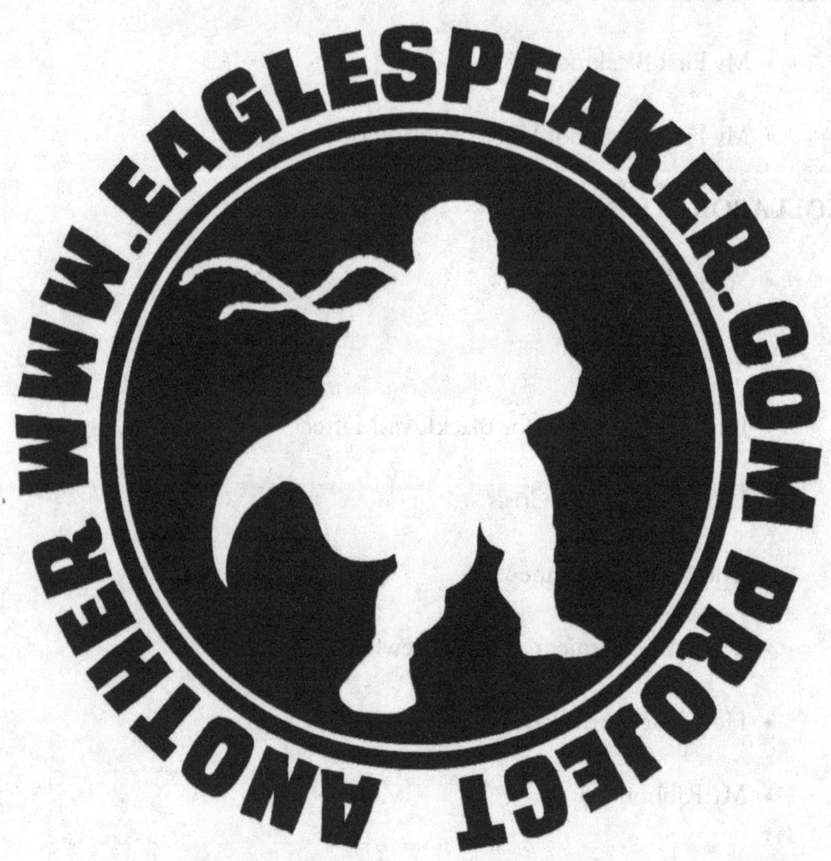

If you loved this book, be sure to find it on Amazon.com and leave a quick review.
Your words help more than you realize.

Be sure to check out plenty more authentically Indigenous publications at
eaglespeaker.com

1. Kuns'i maka (pronounced Koohn – shee – mah – kah): means "Grandmother Earth" in Dakota language

2. Dakodiapi (pronounced dah-koh-dee-yah-pee): means "Dakota language"

3. C'anku Duta (pronounced chahn-koo Doo-tah): means Red Road, sober living, sobriety journey while embracing Dakota traditions in Dakota language

4. Uns'ica (pronounced oohn-shee-kah): Dakota for down on your luck, in need, pitiful

5. Kuns'i (pronounced koohn – shee): Dakota for grandmother/grandma

6. Tiwah'e (pronounced Tee-wah-heh): Dakota for family within one's household

7. Watec'a (pronounced wah-teh-chah): Dakota for leftover food, to-go food, food to take home.

8. Ohiya (Pronounced Oh-hee-yah): means "win" in Dakota language.

9. Dakota C'aje (pronounced Dah-Ko-dah Cha-jay): and means Dakota name

10. Hunk'a (pronounced hoohn-kah): Dakota for adopted, non-blood relative

11. Tanyan aye kte (pronounced Tahn-yahn-ah-yeh-k'teh): the belief that things will work themselves out, in a good way in Dakota language.

12. Bdeh'imic'iye (pronounced ba-deh-hee-mee-Chee-yeh): means strength comes from within, the ability to strengthen thy self, in Dakota language.

9 798359 655897